CONDOMS, BRAS AND STRAIGHTJACKETS

The Young Man's Guide to Female Management

by

Charles A. Becker and William S. Brannigan, Jr

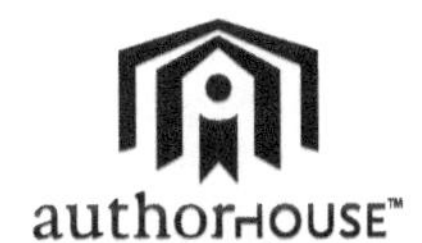

1663 Liberty Drive, Suite 200
Bloomington, Indiana 47403
(800) 839-8640
www.AuthorHouse.com

First published by AuthorHouse 07/08/05

ISBN: 1-4208-1543-1 (sc)
ISBN: 1-4208-1544-X (dj)

Printed in the United States of America
Bloomington, Indiana

This book is printed on acid-free paper.

TABLE OF CONTENTS

CHAPTER 1

WHY READ THIS SHIT?

There was an old man who was considered to be the wisest in this small community. A group of younger men approached him and questioned him. "Old man, how did you get to be so wise?" The old man replied "Good experiences". The younger men asked, "Old man how do you get good experiences?" The old man grinned and replied, "bad experiences".

Why would you spend the time, (and the money), to read this book? Men typically don't "read" self-improvement books. Women typically do that because they're still not happy with their life, and can't understand why, (which is why they're constantly searching for an answer). Typically when men read it usually has to do with hunting, sex, fishing, sex, sports, sex, NASCAR, naked women, killing shit, sex, and maybe a little sex. Maybe it's time "we" did some reading for improvement of the male species. Books have a tendency to pass on successes and/or mistakes in hope that the reader will gain some knowledge and avoid some of the pitfalls that were made by others. Maybe by reading our "bad and good" experiences you can gain some wisdom without going through what we had to.

STRANDED IN THE UDAIRI

This book is a product of the off duty hours of two Army officers during the Second Gulf War. We had just arrived at Camp Wolf, Kuwait when we drove into the Udairi desert. I watched with awe the combination of the desolation and beauty of our new environment. Our unit arrived at Camp Udairi, Kuwait during a heavy sand storm. It was hard to see, but I felt that once the storm abated we would be all right. To my dismay instead of seeing soldiers "hunkered" down waiting for the end of the storm, they were outside going about their business, playing basketball and weightlifting. All of a sudden I realized, there was no storm, it was just Udairi, our "home" for the next year. I leaned over to my buddy and said we are so, so fucked! My friend looked at me with a look of sadness mixed with resolution and said you are so right. This isn't uncommon for us, we're well trained in the art of being fucked. We had both been married and divorced.

After completion of our duty day there wasn't much to do in Udairi. So without the benefit of a TV or a fireplace, we sat around and talked a lot with our fellow officers and soldiers. We had quickly exhausted all the traditional subjects, (sex, sports, naked women, sex, hunting, sex, fishing, sex and killing shit etc…). Eventually we started to talk about our women, bitches and babes, past and present. What came out of those talks was a theme reoccurring so many times in my own life and my buddy's. My friend and I continued to talk about our losses and the penalties of loving women. My friend had wasted 17 years of his life of love, youth and a good part of his ambition on one woman. I chose to spread mine evenly among three. The end result was the same, we were divorced, poor and any hope of our early retirement went out with the "rap" of the judge's gavel.

What was interesting was we didn't classify ourselves as "fuck sticks". Neither of us had the typical asshole traits that traditionally ended relationships. We weren't womanizers, abusers, gamblers, drank to excess, do drugs, or were control freaks. So why were we plagued with ungrateful, unappreciative and worthless women who's greatest contribution to society was changing food into shit?

The military had taught us to perform what's called "after action reviews" on any operation after its completion. It's kind of a militarily sponsored self-actualization program. We decided to apply it to our own lives in the hope to not make any more mistakes. After long hours of our "after action review", we determined that we weren't "fuck sticks" as our wives thought. We had just CHOSEN our women unwisely. At the time of our choosing we didn't have the wisdom we now possessed. In retrospect we wondered how could we have been so blind?

THE NEW WORLD ORDER

What has happened in America was the dawning of a "New world Order", ushered in through the changing sexual mores, (meaning that shit has changed and women give it up really easy now) and the women's liberation movement. For the men we assumed that we were still playing by the "old rules" while the women, (and the courts) basked in the sun of this "new world order". Since the sexual revolution came and went the old rules were tossed away and no new education provided to men. We were still stuck in the same old cultural quagmire of our fathers. This culture was that of John Wayne. When Maureen O'Hara would get out of line John would grab a small hand shovel and spank her in the middle of the town square, (watch the movie "McClintok"). She'd rub her sore ass, go home and everything would be all right. This ideology might have worked for our fathers and Grandfathers, but it's failing miserably for us, (hence the 50% divorce rate).

OUR GOAL

We, (men in general), haven't the slightest insight into the management of women today. Even in the oldest tribal cultures, the young men were given at least a rudimentary education of the opposite sex. Today no one has bothered to give out the rules because they were being made and changed on a day-by-day basis.

The goal of this book is to provide the necessary insight to the man in order to keep his head above water. The rules change at break neck speed but we've found that there are certain truths that will give the man enough information to formulate a plan for survival. Survival is defined as the ability to AVOID those women that would lead him astray from a full rewarding life. And to find the right woman that will allow him to be committed, raise a family and live the "American dream". This will enable him to once again become the leader of our societal family unit as he travels through the uncharted territory of the new world order.

THE FISCAL BREAKDOWN OF LOVE

Divorce in America is right around the 50%, (43-52% in various studies). That simply means one out of every two marriages will end up in divorce. Second marriages fail around 63%, (two out of three), and the percentage increases for every marriage after that. The odds aren't good guys we now live in the "New World Order" and we can't change it back.

To maximize your chances, you have to be right on the first time to have any hope at all at a decent life. The courts now actually make it easy and beneficial for a woman to divorce.

During the marriage ceremony, we stand in front of the alter gazing at the symbols of the most holiest of holies. We make a spiritual, mental and now most recently a long-term financial commitment to a woman. We commit to this woman that statistically has a 50% chance of financially thrashing our ass severely in years to come. Do you really think we like to do it that way? No! Typically men don't like to have their life savings slashed in half, exorbitant monthly dues to have children that you can only see once and awhile, and generally end your early retirement dreams because you're poor as a fucking bag lady. Men simply would like the women they fell in love with to stay and honor their agreements. Men who marry typically want commitment with the right woman.

A typical divorce can run from $2,500 – the sky's the limit. Once in court and the lawyers are on autopilot, you can spend $750.00 in lawyer's fees to "win" a set of golf clubs that might bring $200 in the classifieds. A typical "settlement" could run like this:

1) Community property will net her 50% of your marital assets. "Marital assets" defined is anything that is acquired by you or your spouse during the period you married. Houses, cars, stocks, bonds, bass boats, guns, businesses and retirement plan are up for grabs. This is pretty much a given in most states. i.e. If you have a house for 10 years and it's equity is worth $60,000 then you owe her $30,000. Or she can keep your house and she'll either sell it when the kids are grown and give you your half then or buy you out. The real nice part is when you pick your children up at "your house" and it also houses another man, (sucks to be you).
2) Child support. States differ on child support but a good rule of thumb is 20% of your net for the first child, 25% for two and it slowly gets larger for each successive child. Example: If you have two children and make $50,000 a year you can expect to pay around $900-$1,000 a month, (think of the house, car or boat you could buy for that type of money). Also think about how the loss of that money will hurt you in your life. Additionally, if you make more money you'll be expected to pay more child support. This is a never ending process. Overtime, second jobs and anything that is reported on your income tax is counted.
3) Insurance. Typically the man has to pay for the insurance of the child and maintain a life insurance policy on himself made payable

to his ex-wife. He's also responsible for ½ of the co-pay medical bills.

4) College. When the child turns 18 does the child support stop? Wrong Skippy. Most divorce settlements can include some sort of monetary support through college, (plus ½ the tuition). So work very, very hard, (but not too hard, because she can take you back to court for increased monetary support).
5) Alimony. Notice that the root word here is "money". Many states will give the woman alimony for a period of years. This can be called "recuperative alimony" which lasts for a period of years to get her "back on her feet", or just because they think she needs it. It can be based on her current income potential. Whatever the case it can be up to an additional 20% of your income.
6) Pensions. We live in an uncertain world. The US government is seriously considering changing Social Security and the corporate environment is trending towards markedly reducing or eliminating their pension plans. Note United Airlines' revelation of it's underfunded pension plan by 9.8 billion dollars. Frankly the odds aren't good, last year 192 pension plans failed. 40% of the corporations in the 1980s offered pension plans. Today it's closer to 20% and getting worse. Bottom line. You have only yourself to rely on for a survivable retirement. So your ability to choose and maintain a partner will be crucial. You can't afford to give up ½ of your only retirement plan, (unless of course you do like to eat cat food!).

These are the general biggies regarding the costs of a failed marriage. If you happen to get a woman pregnant you can expect to pay at least child support, insurance and collage support. Have we got your attention yet?

IS THIS A HATE BOOK?

After reading so far you might think "Do we hate women?" Absolutely not!!! Sometimes though, the truth will be a little painful to hear without taking great offense, (especially if a woman reads it... duh). We are for lack of a better term "realists" within this "New World Order". We admit to our mistakes, pay our debts of failed love and wish to share our experiences with others in hopes they won't make the same ones we made. It's that simple.

Do we hate skanky, nasty ass bitches that can't commit and fuck up men's lives? Not really, but we certainly don't fucking like'em either, we just want to avoid them. Finding a good woman that has the same level of commitment and love will create a true team, the combination of the two potenticiating their situation. This means that the end result of the two working together is greater than the sum of them working separately. Which is one of the reasons we love women, everyman should have 6 or 7, (just joking).

We would have liked to remain with one woman for the rest of our lives. But we listened to the promises of the women we loved and got trashed. Like the sailors of old who listened to the sirens of the surf, we were drawn to the rocks and crashed. We still believe in committed relationships and probably will end up in one eventually. We just will be much more discriminating in our future choices.

WHY MARRIAGE?

With the odds sucking so badly why be married in the first place? Marriage is taking a biological stranger and turning that person into your closet relative. Regardless of what most men say, the majority of men will marry at least once. A man will meet a woman who makes him feel a certain way and whammo! He's walking down the isle whistling zippidy do dah out of his asshole. Men are driven to procreation If for nothing else than to obtain some level of immortality by passing a snipit of their genetic material to their offspring. This book has three objectives:

1) To help you choose a woman that will give you the best chance of success for your plan. This will include helping you develop a plan for yourself and incorporating your prospective mate into it.
2) To help you avoid those women who are detrimental to you and your plan. We want to help you identify and avoid those women who are "Never really truly happy", mentally unstable and emotionally scarred or just plain scary.
3) Once you have selected and committed to your mate we'll show you tips on how to maintain that relationship for the duration of your lifespan. Even if you find the "right girl" you still have to nurture the relationship. If you neglect it then there's always a future "fuck-stick" out there who'll will listen to her "problems" to steal her away or just "borrow her" for a while. It will also help you in establishing the "Alpha-Dog" leadership/management position that you need to be successful.

GENERAL MARRIAGE FACTS

Here are some general observations regarding the benefits of marriage vs. single or divorced life:

1) Lifespan. Married men have a 20% greater chance of living to 65 years of age over their single or divorced counterparts. When you live in a stable, loving and supportive relationship you have less stress, more stable living conditions etc.
2) Wealth. Married couples have a national average net worth of $133,000 vs. $33,000 for single/divorced men. Most women work. If you're in a relationship where you don't have to give up 25% of your net income to her and she can donate her income to the family, you naturally will have more money. Also when you're single you're going to have to have sex. Pussy costs money, (at least to maneuver it into position). So again your overall disposable income is less.
3) Child development, Judith Wallerstein notes in her book, "The Unexpected Legacy of Divorce", the following:
    a. Missing role models. Adult children of divorce lack pictures of a healthy marriage partnership. Children from intact families take strength from their parents' marriages. Even the choice to stay in an unhappy marriage. "Just because the adults are unhappy does not mean the children are. No matter how you look at it or spin it the children are always affected. This is especially true when they meet mommy's new "biker boyfriend", (or biker girlfriend).
    b. Prolonged adolescence. When children of divorce provide emotional support to wounded parents, as they often do, bonds are harder to break.
    c. A diminished shot at life. The fathers of 90% of the children with intact families contribute to college expenses. Fewer than 30% of the children of divorce receive help from them. This is true since the combined income of Mom and Dad working is lost, and the father is paying for the children's support and his own.
    d. Rough step family relations. Remarriage shifts a parent's efforts to pleasing a new spouse, at least at the start. Of the 67% of children in Wallerstein's study who grew up with divorce and remarriage of one or both parents, only a fraction bonded with all members of the blended families.

e. More at "risk" behavior. The children of a divorce use drugs and alcohol before age 14 more often than do the children of intact families. Girls have earlier sexual experiences. Is fucking guys early and doing drugs what you want your daughter to do? She'll be the bell of the ball with the guys.
f. Less social competence. A reported 67% of the children of divorce rated above average in competence of work, but only 40% functioned well in social relationships. Another 33% went to therapists to work through their personal lives.

If you examine it, getting married and having children carries not only an emotional weight, but also a financial and even a generational consequence to it. Which is why you want to really take your "best shot" at finding a partner.

This book is addressed to the brave lads who dare to start a relationship in this new world order. A guide for an enigma known as the woman. It is a down and dirty, straight forward, bottom line up-front publication. It's written by two average guys whose education and emotional sins have been paid for with blood, sweat and tears... oh yeah and lots and lots of cash too. We don't have sophisticated theories to state or quote, but we believe that we can offer our "street smarts" sufficiently to the many "regular guys" out there.

The next two chapters are "meaty" and you need to understand this mental "alphabet" that's explained in them. Once through these chapters you'll travel fast and begin to understand our point.

Throughout this book the reader will see some military terms, (sorry but that's our thing). They're used in humorous situations and should be self-evident to the reader. We try to tell our tale in an upbeat humorous way. We curse, make sexist insinuations and generally talk like we're in the locker room, the fishing boat or around a campfire on the Udairi frontier. The traditional boring highbrow PhD's theories, Bill Clinton I feel your pain, and Shirley McClain out on a limb shit won't be seen in this book. We're not writing literature here we're prescribing "male salvation". This is a survival book for the male species. We're not rearranging the deck chairs on the Titanic, we tell you what we think you need to save the fucking boat! This is our story...

CHAPTER 2

THE NATURE OF A WOMAN

A long time ago, men and women existed in roles that hadn't changed since the dawn of time. Each sex fit into a general mold, a design inspired by God himself, a particular cog in the machine we called life.

HISTORY

During WWII, the United States went to war. We won the war but lost something in our American culture. The war and the shortage of manpower necessitated the use of women in what could be called traditional male roles. Once women had found out that they could perform practically the same jobs as men, the world as America knew it no longer existed. It broke longstanding beliefs and forever established rituals regarding the roles of men and women.

During the 1960s, two defining moments occurred for the markedly changed status of women. One was the advent of the birth control pill. The other was the arrival of Betty Friedan.

Birth control released women from the bondage of motherhood. Just as Colt with his revolver made all men equal, the pill made all men and women equal in the bedroom. Prior to this event, women were imprisoned by their role as baby maker and mother. Eventually, regardless of the qualifications of the woman, pregnancy would route the woman out of the workplace and into the home. Women, with the pill, now had a "choice" with regards to procreation.

After this new freedom emerged, Betty Friedan wrote a book entitled The Feminine Mystique. Her book basically described the role of women in the U.S. and asked the burning question, “Is that all there is?” Women and women’s media inhaled this book, and its concepts spread throughout the nation. It should be noted that Betty Friedan initially wrote on women’s issues in the late 1940s, starting with a pamphlet for the American Communist Party.

HOW DID THIS HAPPEN

What fueled this realization for women to “have it all”? As stated earlier, women experienced the dual role in the 1940s. The 1950s allowed family units to experience a greatly accelerated standard of living because of the second income that women produced. The nicer house, vacation homes, and regular new cars validated the woman in the workplace. In the 1960s, the pill and Betty Freidan ushered in the first major break in traditional female values.

During the 1970s and 1980s, the single female parent was validated in the courts. Currently women, on the surface, can literally “have it all.” She can marry, have children, and if she decides to get divorced, she can enjoy approximately 25 percent of her spouse’s net income. She can have half the family savings, home, and retirement fund. Post divorce, she has a baby-sitter every other weekend and help with the finances when it’s college time. All this and still a façade of a weak, helpless victim in the eyes of American society (and, of course, the divorce judge). With this type of situation, the female has a significant “safety net” if she’s not happy with her man. In some cases, it’s almost beneficial for her TO get a divorce. Do you see why whom you pick is so important?

THE INNER CONFLICT

As women achieved the “male goals” they coveted so much, we still find them asking, “Is that all there is?” Even though they have thrown off the bonds of unplanned children, the drudge of marriage, and discrimination in the workplace of the man’s world, they still can’t shake off the yoke of their own genetic makeup. Women by nature are nurturers, mothers, and generally the caregivers of the human species. Society may change, time may change, and technology may change, but women will never change. Career vs. motherhood, executive vs. wife. It’s a no-win scenario. No matter what they do or how they act, this conflict will always rage inside them to some degree. We as men must understand this conflict if we are to attempt to understand women. We say attempt because if women still can't figure themselves out, how can we? Managing females is an art or a "practice." There are very few "finites" that men love to have.

Living the multifaceted lives they have sought after throughout the last thirty years has brought them to the same station as their male counterparts. Now they're not only experiencing the same midlife crises that men encounter in their forties, they are also experiencing the sorrow for the lost opportunities of motherhood and family.

THE NATURE OF THINGS

Frederick Winslow Taylor is considered the "father of scientific management." His theories revolutionized the working world. In a nutshell, Mr. Taylor's theories fit into one statement: "If you can define it… you can control it." He would break down an action or process into its smallest functional parts and try to improve on its performance by manipulation of its external environment. In the workplace, this was a revelation that helped to fuel the industrial revolution of our nation.

Keeping Taylor in mind, we want to try and define the "nature of a woman." Do we expect to quantify the essence of a woman's psyche like we would a manufacturing process? No. Since the woman's psyche is very fluid and dynamic, creating a "static picture" isn't really possible. As we said earlier, this is an art without many finite (concrete) values. But there are a few. We believe that there exist certain patterns and truths that are common to all females. We want to detail these patterns and truths to understand the females' thought process. This is in hope that it will give you the necessary insight to decipher her wants and reactions. If we succeed then you won't be thinking your woman is a crazy bitch and she won't think of you as an asshole. Our end-state is peaceful co-existence for a long-term relationship.

The Turtle and the Scorpion. Once upon a time, there was this turtle swimming along the edge of the water of a rather wide stream. A scorpion appeared at the water's edge and politely asked the turtle for a ride to the other side of the stream, for it was critical that he reach the other side. The turtle answered, "No, because you'll sting me and I'll die." The scorpion answered, "That makes no sense; if I do that we'll both die." Reluctant, but realizing the logic in the scorpions answer, the turtle agreed. At mid-stream, the turtle felt a sting in his neck and as he began to lose control of his muscles and slip below the water's surface, he asked the scorpion, "Why did you sting me? Now we're both going to die." The scorpion answered, "Because it's in my nature."

This little story is necessary. It reinforces the fact that most women will eventually "act their nature." Regardless of promises, contracts, and coercion, they will revert to their natural state eventually or under stress. It's important that you determine the nature of the woman that you have selected. This nature is maintained in two categories: the first of which is likely to be common to all women, while the second category is specific to the one woman you have focused on. The objective here is to never forget the potential nature of women in general. This can be offset by her particular nature, but those actions generic to the sex are always present in some form or another.

THE POSTULATES

In our experiences we have discovered several feminine "truths." Like geometry, we choose to call them the "postulates," for we believe them to be rock-solid truths. This is from the Latin postulatus, to assume or claim as true, existent, or necessary. Postulates are beyond question and considered un-challengeable. We believe that women can ignore these postulates for short periods of time, but they'll eventually surface and have to be "dealt with." Whenever the female is under stress, she can (and frequently does) return to her "default" programming. This is why it's so important to understand the postulates. As we progress in the book, we will list new postulates.

FORGIVE AND FORGET

This will introduce the first of our postulates. The first and most important is POSTULATE #1: "SHE WILL FORGIVE, BUT NEVER FORGET."

Women have an infinite capacity to forgive. It goes along with their innate nurturing and caring ability. It also allows them to continue with paths and decisions that benefit them by allowing them to work through their anger. In nature women are "hardwired" to be the caretakers of the offspring. Because of this, they can't easily run away from a shitty situation. Becoming accommodating (and forgiving) developed in their "nature" as a survival skill not only for themselves but also for their offspring. (Remember, even though she's "hardwired" for certain ideas and concepts, she can still consciously override this default programming). The man must realize that although the woman forgives she will never "forget" the things she forgives. These are written down in some "mental notebook" to be opened years later if need be. It's amazing that even though these transgressions happened years ago, the ink and pages of the mental notebook are crystal clear for the woman. This can apply to your actions or the actions of others. They can be carried from relationship to relationship (old lovers, parents, and friends) into new relationships. Hence the concept of "baggage."

Your (or some other man's) transgressions may have happened years ago, but for her it can be as crystal clear as if it were yesterday. So as you travel along your relationship with a woman, remember that, as with the law, "anything you say or do can and may be used against you in a court of feminine feelings" later.

Actions on the Objective: Review the section on "responsibilities of the alpha leader." Leaders can't be dictators or despots. They have to be concerned with the maintenance of a happy populace (your woman). Always be aware that as the leader, everything you do and everything you say is seen and remembered in some form or another.

THE MENTAL "STAMP BOOK"

Everybody remembers just about everything. It's recorded either consciously or subconsciously. There is a theory regarding a mental stamp book that people maintain in their heads. As they travel through life, they place stamps in the book. Little events that cause stress with no action taken, but that are recorded in their book/mind. Eventually, one day the book is almost filled up. Then some seemingly unimportant event occurs, placing the last stamp in the book. The individual redeems the book at that time, "flipping out" all over the place. Most people have seen this happen in their own lives. The little events are cumulative in that person's mind. As time flows by, they're "added up" and eventually it overloads that person's capacity to compensate.

Why are we detailing this? Most men principally live in a concrete reality. 1 + 1 = 2, right is right and wrong is wrong. Women, on the other hand, tend to live in an "abstract" reality: he said this; I'm going to do this; sexual infidelity vs. emotional infidelity. The problem is that with an abstract thought process, women can equate apples and oranges, allowing anything to be rationalized. We believe that women utilize this concept and the concept of the stamp book to a much greater extent than men do. This leads up to POSTULATE #2: "WHAT YOU SAY AND DO CAN BE USED AGAINST YOU IN THE COURT OF FEMININE FEELINGS."

THE COURT OF FEMININE FEELINGS

The Court of Feminine Feelings. We've used the term earlier. Does it exist? Yes, it does, not in an official, tangible sense, but in a subconscious, unofficial sense. As we discussed earlier, women have a tremendous capacity to forgive. As the couple travels through life the bad (and the good) gets recorded for her posterity. If some emotional event occurs, she has the option to open up this file and the latest session of the court of feminine feelings has started. If you have been a fuck stick and many offenses exist against you and the current offense is serious, then you could be in violation and either punishment or banishment could be ordered. Sometimes the offense isn't critical but mundane or minor. But in the woman's mind, a whole lot of minor can equal a major crime. The man can also get charged for crimes of commission, omission, and alienation of affection (lack of passion). Additional mitigating circumstances can play in the decision as well, i.e., fucked-up childhood, death of a parent, etc.

Example: A female office worker has the following situation: She has been married for almost twenty years. Her parents had divorced when she was sixteen. She had left the house shortly after that, running off with a guy whom she eventually married. The couple eventually had children and she started to realize that her husband spent an enormous amount of time away from the house (the husband was an avid sportsman). During this time, she had grown complacent with his actions. The offenses had built up on the court docket, and eventually the sentence was rendered. She had met a man at her workplace, where she justified herself into having an affair with him, eventually leaving him. After assessing the emotional damage to her children by the breakup, she returned to the husband. She denied her husband having an affair, but felt that she could have one secondary to his crime of unintentional abandonment. Currently, she occupies her time with small affairs with married or unmarried men, still seeing herself as a victim of her husband.

Crimes of the Sex. Another offense that frequently makes it into the court docket is "crimes of the sex." This is not to be considered "crimes of sex." These are two completely different issues. Crimes of the sex are the aggregate crimes of men in "general" that you "specifically" have to answer for. Because you're in the group that happens to have a penis, you'll share in the guilt of that species.

Example: Some man at work has fucked her over at work, probably acting like a man. This pissed her off, but she can't say anything to him. Or some fuck stick (man) has fucked over one of her friends in a relationship, and she can't say anything to him either.

She is distraught about this, and since she can't thump the nuts of the fuck stick that pissed her off, she'll settle for thumping yours. This typically isn't a major offense, but a minor one. Without recognition of the syndrome—POSTULATE #3: "WOMEN TEND TO SHARE THEIR UNHAPPINESS"—you might engage in an argument that could possibly leave you with no sex for a while.

Actions on the Objective: When you recognize the woman's distress, don't just sit there and read the fucking paper. Stop what you're doing and GIVE HER SOME ATTENTION! Nothing needs to be fixed here. She simply needs you to listen to her (don't dare laugh either) and reassure her that everything is going to be all right.

One important note: NEVER ENGAGE IN THE DEFENSE OF THE ALLEGED PERPETRATOR. Occasionally some asshole will feel the need to defend his "species." What typically happens is they fight and he will by proxy assume the fuck stick's guilt. It will be remembered and recorded (See POSTULATE #1). This is pissing into the wind for sure. If she tells you what the fuck stick did then you have two options:

1) Agree with her that the guy was a fuck stick (it's no skin off your ass).
2) Keep your mouth zipped. If you can't agree with her then shut the fuck up.

"EMOTIONAL" BAGGAGE

Since we mentioned it, we should discuss it. Keeping in mind our newest postulate, we have to discuss "baggage" and its relationship to POSTULATE #1: "SHE WILL FORGIVE BUT NEVER FORGET."

If you are fortunate enough to date a woman who has never had anything bad happen to her then consider yourself a very lucky bastard. But those of us who tend to live in the real world need this advice. Most women (and some men) have a certain amount of emotional baggage. Emotional baggage is the bad experiences that people carry in their mind/emotions from the past that persist from relationship to relationship (some examples are child abuse, substance abuse, and/or crazy ex-partners). Even though you didn't do it, if you "trigger" the memory you will experience at least some of the pain of the event.

War Story. Jim was enjoying sex with his relatively new girlfriend Kathy. Kathy was dripping hot and the sex was top-shelf. During a hot point, Jim slipped his finger into one of Kathy's unauthorized orifices in hopes to bring her to a higher high. Well, he apparently pulled the "stop cord" of her "O" train, for she came to a screeching halt (neither of them made it to the station that night). After several days of "talking it out," she had apparently had a physically, sexually abusive relationship with a guy a few years prior to Jim. It had involved a lot of back-door action that had left her with some "baggage." Eventually Kathy and Jim worked out their differences and moved on with their relationship. It took Jim a while to get Kathy back to the level of sexual performance she had once been at. Was Jim the sexually, physically abusive guy? No, but he did pay for that other guy's sin, to a lesser degree. And, of course, he never touched or mentioned the "back door" again.

This is an example of "minor emotional baggage." It wasn't considered major and was, with a small amount of time, resolved. They're other types of baggage, which we will address later.

SHARING

Women have a tendency to telegraph their feelings. Typically when a person is happy, they like to share it with others. Men do this as well, but women like to share unhappiness. Men typically don't do this. When unhappy, men tend to go to their fortress of solitude and try to think of a way out of whatever made them unhappy. When a woman is unhappy, she typically can't tolerate her mate being happy (happy to a woman can be the absence of unhappiness). So they will act in certain ways to upset the world of the man so that he can attempt to achieve the same level of misery that she has. We now can introduce POSTULATE #3: "WHEN A WOMAN IS UNHAPPY SHE WILL TEND TO PROJECT HER UNHAPPINESS ONTO THE MALE." Now that you're unhappy, she has an unwilling accomplice to her struggle. You will, because you're a man, put on your male hat and try to help her figure out a solution for her problem (or argue with her, if you're stupid). She doesn't want this because that would involve making a decision, and women don't do those well.

Actions on the Objective. When we encounter a problem, we like to give an immediate course of action that could help you in your dilemma. We recommend that you don't try to help the woman out of her situation. What she really wants is to have you hold her, make stupid, soothing noises, and tell her it will be "all right." Now this makes absolutely no fucking sense to us, but it does work eventually. The woman will cycle through her emotions and you will be rewarded for your sensitivity (read: good sex). If she does ask you for specific help then you can give it. But walk carefully, for this is a dangerous area. Give advice but don't take control of the situation (even if you know you can do it quickly and efficiently). We also recommend you read Men are from Mars, Women are from Venus.

This is an excellent book that goes into great detail on the communicative road hazards that females have and how to avoid them.

DECISION MAKING

We have to talk about the female decision-making process. It's always been said that women have different mechanisms of decision making than men. As we have said earlier, their thinking tends to be more abstract and involved than men's. Men by nature are much more concrete thinkers than women. We believe that this difference markedly differentiates the decision-making process between males and females.

This leads us to POSTULATE #4: "WOMEN TEND TO LET SITUATIONS EVOLVE RATHER THAN MAKE A SOLID DECISION." Now don't think that women can't be focused. They can and frequently are more focused than the male. But this isn't their "nature." They tend to make decisions by manipulating their external environment to help the evolution of their situation. To come out and make a decisive change is not typical for them (unless they're functioning as a male).

War Story. Sally was twenty-nine and in a loveless marriage (read: unhappy). She eventually met a man at work and rationalized herself into having an affair. After a while, she decided that she was in love with this man. The only two things that were wrong were that she was still married and so was he. She felt that her world would be complete if she could pursue an open relationship with her lover. But she couldn't come out and make the decision. She couldn't say to her husband, "I want to leave you." So she did the passive-decision process and got really lazy in her infidelity security. She didn't seem to care about getting caught and eventually she did. After a lot of drama, she was free and so was her lover. What we have observed is managed evolution in process. Neither male caught on to what had happened. Men believe in the adage "shit happens." But was it shit happening? Or was it the nature of a woman?

2 + 2 = 4... NOT ALWAYS

In the world of physical sciences and math, we have learned that there are absolutes. If you do this action, then this resultant action will happen. Guys love this shit. We're comfortable in the fact that we could repeat this and it would happen again and again. It was a 100 percent solution. Men are typically concrete thinkers and like our finite thoughts and values.

In the world of female emotion, there isn't an absolute all the time. No 100 percent solution (though they try hard to achieve it). Where men think, women feel. What's an absolute core value today for the female might not be even a close answer tomorrow. Obviously men have been driven to drink because of this. (I guess we had to have some reason for it.) As we travel through the female psyche and emotions we have to keep this postulate in mind. POSTULATE #5: "TWO PLUS TWO DOESN'T ALWAYS EQUAL FOUR." This doesn't mean that women can't be consistent. They can be very consistent... if they want to. The key point here is that they don't HAVE to be consistent. They can switch in and out of this mode without penalty. Men can be inconsistent as well, but they will pay a price for that aberration. They are held to a different standard since they are supposed to be leaders. Leaders have to be consistent.

CONFESSION

Confession is a tool for the woman to absolve herself from any responsibility for her actions. It's a wonderful tool for her because the man (most unlike the woman) has the ability to "forget what he forgives." Yes, it's true. Once a man truly forgives someone of something, it will typically be forgotten after a period of time. So "confession is good for the soul" (if the man forgives).

The problem is that men don't always forgive the things that a woman confesses to. Things like Ethics, Values, and Integrity (EVI) issues are very non-forgiving issues. Like the woman fucking the guy at work. That's a serious EVI issue. She not only let some fuck stick into her most "sacred place," but she probably utilized multiple lies to accomplish the event. Some men will say they forgive the woman, but in reality they don't... period! Where women have the innate ability to forgive, men just simply say, "Fuck it," and move on. They also may say, "Fuck him," and go find the miserable son of a bitch and kick/kill/or maim him. The possibilities are endless. From that time on, the woman in the eye of the man will bear the "scarlet letters" FWB (fucking whoring bitch). No, he might not say it directly to her if he decides to stay, but he will never, ever, ever forgive her completely.

Most women are aware of this EVI clause when it comes to confession and the subsequent lack of total forgiveness. Since they tend to "need" to confess they will develop some form of the following types of confessions. The alpha dog should be aware of these abnormal confessions. They are:

COVERT CONFESSION

The need for a woman to confess is strong. They have to "get it out" and gain the absolution of their partner. This is typically a selfish thing because the woman doesn't realize the pain that's caused by the confession. They could go to a priest, a counselor, or of anyone with anonymity. But to a woman, it isn't the same as gaining absolution from the offendee.

We believe that the incentive a woman uses to confess centers around two general areas:

1) I need to confess because I'm in danger of getting caught.
2) I need to confess to "cleanse" myself to get on with my life and eventually gain the "moral high ground."

For less serious offenses. When women are in fear of getting caught, they will undoubtedly run to confession in hopes that they can secure absolution (forgiveness) for their sin. They have somehow reasoned that if they confess now and squirt a few tears then the man will assure her it is all right and it can't be THAT bad (i.e., the woman bangs the shit out of the car probably doing exactly the thing the man has told her not to do. The car will eventually be discovered unless she has an "in" with the local body shop. So she will confess, cry about the car, and eventually all will be forgiven).

For more serious offenses. The woman will decide that she must confess, feeling a need to "cleanse" herself. Here are three possible types of confession she might use. They are:

1) The "covert" confession. This is where she will disguise her confession and use a general agreement to gain an absolution for the offense.

   War Story. Dee was dating Carl in a yearlong relationship. Carl was away for a deployment and Dee had gone out and knocked off a piece of ass (women get horny too). Now faced with the need to confess, Dee started on a general-discussion tangent one night regarding physical infidelity vs. emotional infidelity. She was explaining that she didn't feel that physical infidelity was nearly as bad as emotional infidelity. Now, to a man infidelity is infidelity (the dick goes in and it's infidelity; that's it). Carl was trying to figure out where this conversation was going. She didn't gain his agreement on this and it was dropped. Eventually he found out, when it surfaced two years later, that she had been fucking this guy at work while he was gone. She stated it was just a physical thing, but, as you know, guys expect their ladies to behave like a lady, not a fucking slut. Carl had no choice but to dump the bitch.

2) The "tabloid" confession. These types of confessions are intended for servicing the definition of a confession but omitting the most damaging or threatening facts. This is sometime known as the "court" or "plea bargain" confession. Like a tabloid editor or a shyster lawyer, a palatable story on a "sliver of truth" is concocted. It may have some truths about what really happened, but it leaves out the major crime. The woman confesses her "story" to the judge (man) and secures absolution for a lesser offense.

   War Story. James was a good husband who provided a good home for his wife and two children. He was active in church and his children's school. Eventually his wife became "bored" and lonely with the family thing. She eventually pined about her lot in life and sought out an extramarital affair with an employee. After a while, she found out that this avenue didn't provide her happiness and ended the affair. Now at this point she had executed the perfect crime. HE didn't have a clue as to her infidelity. But almost to a day after the affair ended, she confessed. What was interesting was that she didn't confess everything to her husband. Her confession detailed her actions to seeing a man and kissing, feeling up, and everything but penetration. This was bad, but his wife knew that her husband wouldn't tolerate her fucking some other guy. She knew him well enough to leave that major fact out of the confession. And it worked for a while, until the other man became consumed with the loss of "his girl" and called the house, forcing a telephone confrontation. After the new facts came to light, she confessed and the marriage eventually ended.

3) The "blanket" confession. This confession is where the woman will attempt to forgive her partner of all his misgivings if he will in turn forgive her. Nothing specific is stated, but absolution is granted and the woman will feel better, ready to assume the moral high ground.

   War Story. Jane was married for fourteen years to Bob, a decent guy and a good husband. But she developed a severe drinking problem. Eventually, while out drinking three times a week, she developed an affair. (Big fucking surprise, right?) As an obvious reaction, her marriage to Bob was on the rocks. She finally got her head out of her ass, quit the drinking, and ended the affair. But because of her strict Catholic background, she needed to confess and gain absolution for her transgressions. During a marital discussion she offered up a confession in the form of "I'll forgive you of all of your stuff and you forgive me of mine." On the outside, Jane was doing a blanket confession to an obviously lesser offense. In reality, she's getting a blank check to cover ALL her actions. In her mind and reality, she had been absolved of all her wrongdoing. The lies, the excessive drinking, and, of course, all the times she was fucking other guys is (in her mind) forgiven. Was Bob aware of this? He knew something had happened, but he didn't look hard and chose "mushroom status" because of his children.

Actions on the Objective. Your actions are dependent on your goals. Do you want the truth? Or would you rather take "mushroom status" (that means stay in the dark, lying in shit)? Accepting the statement that "men can never really forgive" could make a man choose to leave the situation "undiscovered." This must be your decision not ours. Our job is to make you aware of what might be happening. Always remember that once a woman cheats in a relationship, she will be more likely to do so again.

THE MORAL HIGH GROUND

Women have as an innate intelligence the desire to obtain the "moral high ground" of any given situation. When watching women, it becomes apparent that they "need" the moral high ground. It appears to be one of the constituents of happiness for them.

In their attempt to maintain the moral high ground, they have to manipulate their situation to rationalize their actions. Because of POSTULATE #5: "TWO PLUS TWO DOESN'T ALWAYS EQUAL FOUR," they can pretty much rationalize any action they choose to do. Now, men like to rationalize as well. But we rationalize as a sanity check. Where women do this to a lesser extent, they rationalize for right vs. wrong. Men rationalize to check "does this make sense or not?"

When women weigh their actions, they have very few rules. Since 1) they tend not to make decisions and choose to let something "evolve"; and 2) since they feel instead of think, they can equate anything they want to.

In our world, men can't add apples and oranges. But in the women's world, they sometimes can and frequently do.

Example: A woman can "feel" she's neglected at home. Her husband doesn't talk to her like she thinks he should, he forgets a holiday, or some other shit. After a while she meets a co-worker and feels "justified" into having an affair. Now, her husband didn't have an affair on her, but she can feel completely justified in fucking the guy at work. Women can come up with all sorts of reasons to do whatever they want to do.

Example: Another man's wife maxed out their credit cards when she went away on a vacation. Her reasoning was she got into a fight with her friend at their church. The guy was away on a two-week military mission. When he called his family to talk, she had told him she was packing. She said, "I have to get away. I lost my whole support system." He told her that he would be home in a few days and they could work this out together. She wouldn't hear of it. She had painted this picture of her total world coming apart. And everything of importance lay in the balance of her taking a trip back home. It didn't matter that she had just gotten the house of her dreams and they had no disposable money. It didn't bother her that she stole her stepson's money and maxed out their credit cards. It didn't matter that he would miss his daughter's fifth birthday. What she wanted to do was take a trip home. To her the facts weren't important so long as they supported the truth.

So women can justify practically any action they really want to. The ones with real moral character tend not to do that. Again we emphasize that time is everything. The longer you wait before commitment, marriage, and eventually children, looking over and examining your mate, the better your chances at observing unacceptable behavior.

PHYSIOLOGICAL EFFECTS

The following are some "physiological" characteristics that can influence the psyche of the woman. The effects are real but not an "absolute" for all women. Some are affected partially and others have every fucking symptom. This is a short list of the "potentials." It can be all, part, or none with regards to the effects on the psyche.

HORMONES AND LUNA

There is a topic that must be covered. Sometimes women frequently change their beliefs secondary to hormonal deficiencies and surges. The concept of "rainy days and Mondays always bring me down" can be a real situation. A woman can have a case of the "Mondays" on Tuesday, Wednesday, or any other day. Without getting into a discussion on female hormone physiology, suffice it to say that the "abnormal" level of a woman's hormones can cause wide swings in her personality and mood.

The Effects of the Lunar Cycle. The "lunar cycle isn't something left by the astronauts on the moon. It's the cyclic effects on earth caused by the phases of our moon. The tides are affected by the gravitational pull of the moon. These effects can also affect the smooth operation of some people's minds (and especially some women's actions). If you doubt this, ask anyone who's worked and hospital ER or in a prison on a full moon. Some women are very susceptible to the hormone changes and lunar cycles. If you happen to be dating a female like this, observe the swings of her mood with relation to her period and the full moon. If they're severe, you should look deeper. These typically get worse with the passage of time, not better.

PREMENSTRUAL SYNDROME

Since we've been talking about the effects of hormones on the emotional and mental state of the female, we have to address premenstrual syndrome, more commonly known as PMS. In some cases, mentioning this word causes shivers in full-grown men. Because, in a sense, this is a license for the woman to act anyway she wants to without accountability. Since its identification and the large amount of media given to it, women have had carte blanche in their actions. In the old days, women were held to higher standards of behavior than they are today. If they were suffering then they did so in silence, feeling that to "flip out" was evidence of poor upbringing. Like the hormonal woman above, pay close attention to the female just prior to her period. If she "swings" way out of control then look deeper.

War Story. This is a report from a woman describing her PMS. About one week prior to her period, she gets the following symptoms:

1) Excessive overreaction to minor stimuli (she gets real bitchy and has a short temper). Crying over anything is possible.
2) Clingy. The woman can be extremely clingy and need excessive amounts of TLC.
3) Breast enlargement. You would think this would be a good thing. But it isn't. The breast enlarges possibly due to water retention or the hormonal thing. Bottom line: the breast is tender as hell, adding to her discomfort.
4) Water weight. As her period approaches, she will start to retain water. Gaining weight starts to screw with her "chi" since this is the most sensitive of the "body image" constituents. A woman can easily gain five pounds overnight.
5) Hunger. During this time, the female can be almost perpetually hungry. This, of course, contributes to the weight gain, making her even more unpleasant.
6) Cramps and back pain. This can be almost debilitating according to some females. Hot packs and massage by a nice mate can help.

7) Increased sexual drive (read: horny). Just prior to her period starting, the female gets extremely "ready" for sex (horny). So if you're around, you'd better get it now. Some women don't like their man "shooting the red rapids."
8) Acne. Some women, because of the change in hormones, experience acne, already adding to her temporary self esteem attack.

These are some of the potential symptoms that some women experience. It's uncomfortable, painful for some, and challenging for others. Some women have nothing; others have every fucking symptom. Others don't have shit but say they do for attention or an excuse to get out of unpleasant thing. (Do you think ALL those girls had their period in gym class every week?) If you're interested in why this happens, get a physiology book.

Actions on the Objective. The thing to remember is that you need to feign understanding and give lots of care to the female during this period (no pun intended). If your female is really most sincerely experiencing PMS then she's probably miserable. Remembering POSTULATE #1: "SHE WILL FORGIVE, BUT NEVER FORGET," then you had better be Mr. Fucking Sensitive. Write the week off and collect points for "your time." If you determine that you can't deal with her monthly temporary psychosis then dump her. This type of thing typically doesn't get easier as she gets older (except after menopause).

THE CAMEL TOE CHRONICLES

There is a power that women possess; they like to call it the "power of a woman." Like Satan it is known by many names, "the camel toe, the bearded clam, the gash that never heals." The list can go on and on. Most men tend to call it the power of the "pussy." Regardless of its name, it's heaven on earth for us and a control mechanism that women use.

Women aren't born with the knowledge or power. It's slowly introduced to them through time and society. Remember when we were young? Girls were gross, had "cooties," and if they touched you it was an affliction. As time wore on, these girls got breasts, periods, hips, and asses. They began to enjoy the affections of boys, the competition for their return affection, and the eventual all-star wrestling matches that happen in backseats of cars. It didn't take them long to see the power the class slut possessed. But however long it took, they all eventually found out and started to put it to use to their benefit.

Sam Kinnison humorously discussed this concept in a comedy routine in the 80s. The power of the "pussy." Sam would discuss attending a party and partying a little too hard. His wife gets pissed off and tells him she wants to go. He tears into her, verbally ripping shreds of meat off of her. She waits a beat and says, "I have the pussy." At that point Sam would scream in anguish and tell his buddies goodbye. His only excuse was "she's got the pussy, guys ... she's got the pussy." The other men understood they too were the slaves of the camel toe. This sounds funny but it's not intended to be. History has proven it time and again.

The power that women hold has men doing all sorts of things they never would normally do. Helen of Troy: did Ulysses really want to spend ten years fighting Troy when he could have been playing the Greek equivalent of golf? The face that launched a thousand ships—more appropriately, the pussy that launched a thousand ships. In one classic movie, Anna of a Thousand Days, one of King Henry's council members stated, "The future of France was maintained between the legs of a woman." Mata Hari, one of the most famous female spies: did she use special James-Bond, high-tech instruments? No, she was on her back and extracted countless military secrets from her lovers. Whole countries have been made and destroyed for a very small patch of personal real estate.

If you don't think the camel toe has that much power then look at Gary Hart. He was a "sure thing" for the Democratic presidential challenge, but his actions with Donna Rice on the yacht Monkey Business cost him that. Recently a well-known, married basketball star was plagued by the press and the courts for his alleged sexual actions with a girl in a hotel. The cost? A Nike ad contract ($2-3 million), possible divorce, possible jail time, and possible civil suit. Just the lawyer's fees are probably staggering. Men have paid dearly for it. Women have it and we want it... badly. It's that simple, and there's no effective counter for this sometimes weapon. Men have to accept it, but with early female management and a whole lot of will power, you can lessen its influence in your life.

Actions on the Objective. The first thing we must do in the relationship is convince the woman that the pussy isn't all that! A hard task, but doable. This must take place at the initial dating level. When at first dating, don't go after the pussy immediately, right off. Sex should be consensual and mutual. Remember, you're the leader, you're setting the tempo. However, we know what tempo you'd really want to set. "Hi, I'm here to take you out for a date. Let's fuck before we eat." This obviously isn't good; she'll categorize you with all the "other" men, and she will figure out your addiction for the pussy. You have to be different, march to the beat of a different drummer, take the road less traveled, or other shit like that. You don't really have to be that way; just let her think you're that way. Take her out, wine her and dine her, and let her think she's setting the sexual tempo. Making a move toward the pussy is like looking at the dark side of the force: it will forever control your destiny.

THE POWER OF NO

To enable us to have control, we as men have only one tool in the box. That's the power of no. It's all we have to adequately counter the power of the camel toe. To establish the alpha-dog leadership, we have to set the tempo from the start. We choose when we have sex, which involves waiting and saying no to her until it's at a time of our choosing. Utilizing this in the beginning will repay itself many times in the future. This is only to be used with potential mates. If you're out sport fucking then whatever your style you choose is adequate.

Example: I dated this girl named Heidi. She was ten years younger than me (twenty), nice, beautiful, and horny as hell. We went out, danced, and eventually got to the end of the evening. When I dropped her off I wanted a good-night kiss, she wanted a good-night kiss. I told her I enjoyed being with her and wanted to do it again. Then I shook her hand and opened the door for her to leave. This fucked her "chi" all up; it threw her off balance and her momentum, giving me control of the situation. Men do have some control of the pussy. It's the option not to take it, to turn it down, leave it lie. Or would you rather be a mindless, wandering dick, willing to fuck the head of a snake if you could get someone to hold its head open? This is okay if you're just out sport fucking. But for potential mate selection, it's an alpha-dog faux pas, (French for fuck up).

We got together the next week, talking on the phone a few times to let her know I liked her. On our second date, we had dinner at my place; she was definitely motivated and wanting to regain her lost momentum. We were kissing and rubbing and all that other good stuff, then she decided to play coy with her pussy. She talked about us just meeting and all, not sure if we "should." I assured her that while we were kissing and stuff, I would not take advantage of her in a moment of weakness. This was an obvious attempt to control the pussy and, indirectly, me. If I gave in now, I would be giving in all the time. The line was drawn in the sand. As the evening wore on, she wanted me to lose control and take her pussy in a moment of pure passion. I turned down the pussy (not without great effort and pain, because she was really hot) and told her that my word was my bond and all that other noble type of shit. We would have to wait for the next date to "make love," and she should make this decision when she's not "heated." That was my word, and sex was special to me and not to be frivolously done (so much shit). She then tried to make excuses as to why I shouldn't uphold my word. That she would leave and go around the block. Then it would be the "next date" and we could make love. I held firm (no pun intended) and stood my ground. She left but returned the next day at my invitation and had sex on my terms. That relationship ran for about a year until I decided that she wasn't the one for me.

POST-MARRIAGE ADDICTION

If you have been in a relationship for a while and she's already diagnosed you with pussy addiction, then you are semi-fucked. Your choices are limited and painful. What you have to be aware of is the direct pussy approach. The assault starts like this: you're with your girlfriend or wife and you have committed some act of commission or omission. You forgot to chant your mantra of forgiveness quickly enough or the offense was significant. Regardless you're in the "penalty box." The evening comes: bedtime and you reach for her comfort. You suddenly find yourself transported in time to the backseat of your car, trying in vain to score.

She now has your attention, doesn't she? If you're fortunate enough for her to outright tell you what she is pissed about, then you can find out the penalty for your transgressions. If not, you'll have to play detective. The end state of this exercise is the cessation of sex for the night usually. Your choices are as follows:

1. Discuss. Obviously you're at fault for something (even if it's her inadequacy at life). She's unhappy and it's your job to make her happy again. This is typically not a quick-fix course. It will take a day or two to fix. Resolution of her problem is desirable and you must realize for future reference that her problems are your problems. If introspection leads you to fault on your part then by all means accept your guilt, do your penance, and move on with the relationship. Beware of sliding into the beg zone.
2. The long siege. If this is an initial event, you are at a crossroads in your relationship. Succumbing to this tactic will feed the stray cat of future pussy terrorism. The alpha-dog leader would have to wait it out, as hard as it would be. She would have to come to you for the sexual joys.

   War Story. Carl was living with Sandy and he had committed some minor male crime. She had been cool with him for two days, but being young he didn't realize the disruption. When he initiated sex, she rolled over to him and said, "You don't deserve it." Carl was smart, didn't say anything, and went to sleep. This lasted for three weeks, when she finally initiated sex with him.

He said to her, "I still don't think I deserve it," and waited two more weeks. When he initiated sex with her, she readily gave it up. Since that initial pussy terrorism incident, he has experienced no more episodes of that behavior (he did have blisters on his dick from beating off, though).

This was a good step in the alpha-dog leadership principle. But it has to be remembered that it did have a price. She will remember this incident. Always be conscious of the first postulate and the court of feminine feelings.

3. Stoic. Say nothing and pretend there's no issue, hoping she will get over whatever it is that's bothering her. This could set you up for a long siege, a test of sexual wills for which she has the upper hand (see above). Remember POSTULATE #1: "SHE WILL FORGIVE, BUT NEVER FORGET." Beware of sliding into the beg zone.
4. The ultimatum. This can be a very effective strategy because it plays on the woman's fear of being replaced. The man, on notification of the pussy penalty, will issue the ultimatum that if he doesn't get "it" from his partner he will go elsewhere for satisfaction. Our favorite quote for this goes like this: "They may not be handing pussy out like pie, but you don't have the only one," or words to that effect. While this usually gets the ball rolling, the usual caring, giving, and quality sex that you have experienced in the past is replaced by the "duty sex." Sex by duty is not nearly as rewarding as sex by choice and is commensurate to masturbation. While this services a need, the woman is usually filling the stamp book with "asshole points" for you. This strikes at her self-esteem and her sense of self-worth. She'll think that all she is to him is a piece of ass and will act accordingly. This action causes estrangement and retribution. If sex resumes and the relationship appears okay, the man will forget the whole episode. Quoting POSTULATE #1: "SHE WILL FORGIVE BUT NEVER FORGET." She has forgiven you of your initial sin and the sin where you gave her the "gas, ass, or cash, nobody rides for free" speech. But the whole scenario has been recorded. Years may pass, but it can be as fresh in her mind as if it happened yesterday. So use this approach as a silver bullet.
5. Beg. This is disgusting and we have all done when in the sport fucking mode. In a committed relationship this is the last-ditch effort to allow the man to gain sex. If you have to beg to get sex, then don't. It is not an alpha-leadership position, clearly defensive,

and somewhat yellow. You will not only lose your dignity here, but also reinforce her use of pussy terrorism to keep you in line. Before you use this option, pick out which skirt you want to wear while selling your Girl Scout cookies.

The odd thing is, more often than not, she will most likely maintain some vague level of respect for your standing your ground in this way (you'll still be an asshole, but an asshole with integrity).

Referring to the section on arguing, are you planning the campaign while she is focused on the close fight? Stay away from the close fight; look at the big picture and your future with this woman. At any rate, even though the woman has brought this action on by her own actions/words, she'll still feel that she has been the victim. (Like that's news, right?)

CAN'T WE JUST ALL GET ALONG?

To master this initial concept, the man must realize that in dealing with a woman's psyche there are no absolutes, no 100 percent solution, and no congruencies. It's not saying that a woman can't act very stable. Matter of fact, they can and frequently act more stable than the male. This is on "outward" products and on their "singular" output. What we have listed here are some of the potentials of incongruent thought capable from a woman. Even though their product can be superior, it doesn't mean that their mind didn't have tremendous inner turmoil (from a man's point of view) to get there. The best example that illustrates this is an experiment. Men and women were selected for their matching IQs and very similar educational background. They were placed in a Positron Emission Tomography (PET) device (in which you can see the actual functioning of the brain) and requested to perform complex mathematical problems. What they found was that the men and women completed the problems in the same amount of time and with the same correct answers. What was different was that the PET scanner showed that the men solved the problems in a different part of the brain than did the women.

Men and women are different; be aware of that and adjust your expectations and assumptions accordingly. Don't anticipate her actions to your beliefs and rationales. The higher your expectations, the greater your disappointments can be. Women aren't bad; they're just different, and we as the alpha dog need to see through that, understand it, and compensate.

CHAPTER 3

SELF ESTEEM

This is a meaty chapter, but it's essential to understanding and identifying the undesirable female. Throughout our experiences in life we have noticed that self-esteem plays a large part in the development of every human being. Generally speaking anybody with a low self-esteem doesn't do as well as someone with normal self-esteem. Men tolerate it and can continue to work through it the majority of the time, but women appear to suffer badly from it, (it fuck's up their "chi" preventing them from true happiness). In dealing with women we've noticed that self-esteem is especially important. So much so that we've dedicated an entire chapter regarding our concept of self esteem and it's identification of pathological levels in women. We're calling this a CORNER STONE concept, (important shit that you don't want to forget). We're not going to attempt to provide the insight/information that a professional counselor/psychologist would use. That's for the PhD's, MD's and talk show hosts to pontificate on. We want to give the laymen, (that means us working stiffs); the necessary information to determine what might not be "normal". Then if you choose you can research further or take her to get professional help. If we make a mistake we will make it in the "safety zone" rather than risk being wrong.

LIFE IS A HOUSE.

When thinking of self-esteem, think of a house. You have the walls holding everything up. The walls we're especially concerned with are the "load bearing walls". These are the ones that will support the whole second story of the roof. The roof is a metaphor, (a comparison to get a point across) for the woman's self esteem. The walls are those things that contribute to the self-esteem and solidify the structure. You can move the walls, remove the walls but to keep the roof up you have to build other load bearing walls, (or reinforce existing walls to keep the roof from falling). When there isn't enough "load bearing walls in the structure, the roof will sag, crack or in severe cases completely fall down, (resulting in "crazy bitch" actions or a stay in the "HA-HA Hotel"). When attached to a female who has some of these saggy walls we find ourselves as "mental carpenters" involuntarily drafted to "fix" things up. We typically take these jobs because we're men and we love to "fix things", (it's in our nature). Where we get into trouble is when we estimate a simple repair and it ends up with a major construction project requiring much of our time and of course don't forget the money. We can compound the problem when we don't have enough money or time and end up "cobbling" something together.

In many cases the concept of self-esteem and self worth is the center of the woman's "Chi". Self-esteem is the most important item to good mental health. It allows the woman to feel competent and capable. Most importantly it allows the woman to feel "worthy of happiness", (this is important because if she doesn't feel "worthy of happiness" usually no matter what you do you can't make her happy). Two general components of self-esteem are Self-efficacy and Self worth.

Self-efficacy

– Having trust in your mental abilities. Does she have the necessary "smart equipment" to function in her world? In your world? Or is she "not the sharpest knife in the drawer"?

Self respect

– Your inherent value
- Having friendship, love and happiness, (look at friends, family and past relationships if possible)
- Realizing she deserves the respect of others. Does she allow others to "run over her"?

Self-efficacy and self worth are both necessary to have sufficient amounts of self-esteem. Whole libraries are devoted to this subject. So we can't even begin to do it justice with respect to its causes, (they are endless) and the corrections of poor self esteem, (just as endless). What you must remember is the importance of self-esteem/self worth is the center of the woman's psyche and the identification of potentially pathologically low levels of self esteem.

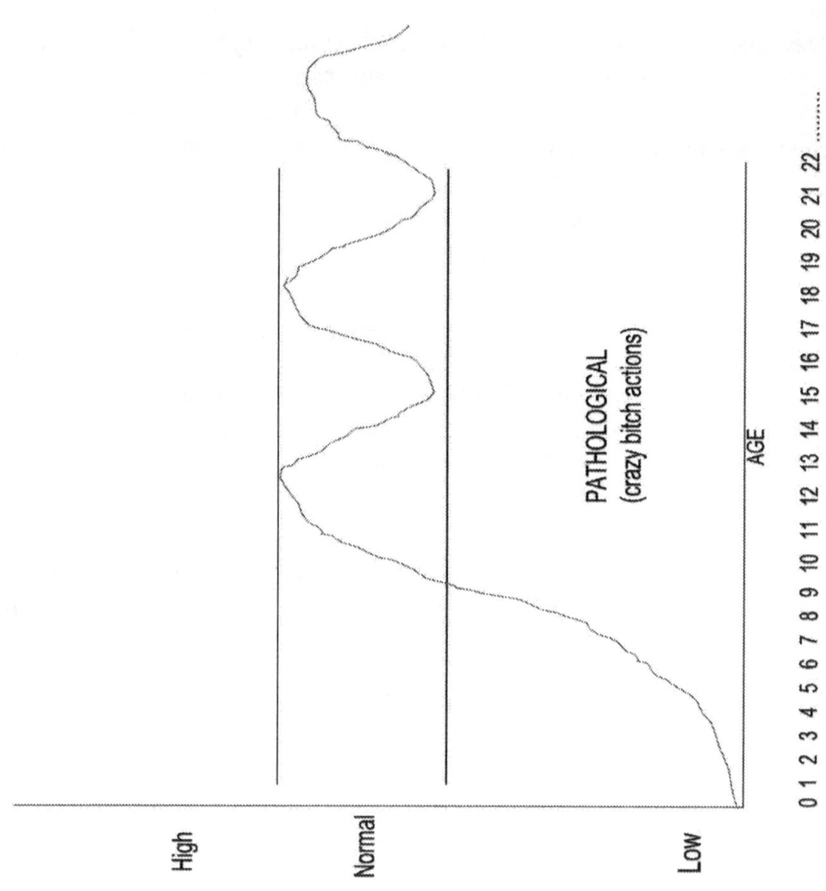
High
Normal
Low
PATHOLOGICAL
(crazy bitch actions)
AGE
0 1 2 3 4 5 6 7 8 9 10 11 12 13 14 15 16 17 18 19 20 21 22 ....

Pathological Self Esteem. What is pathological self esteem? As we look at the diagram above we see a graphic representation of what might happen to a female in a perfect world. At birth self-esteem is probably low. As children we start to develop our self-esteem. As we age we learn, we experience life and eventually gain in self-esteem. In our perfect world there has been only good growth experiences leading to normal development of self-esteem. This is represented by the two horizontal lines, like our body's temperature operates in a range of 92 to 106 degrees. Go above or below that temperature the body ceases to function and damage starts to occur. When a destructive force destroys or lowers the self-esteem into the "pathological zone" we start to see some manifestations of abnormal/destructive behaviors. This is what guys call "crazy bitch" actions, (it's an industry term).

THE UNIFIED "FEELING" THEORY

We believe that the woman's self esteem is similar to Einstein's Unified Field Theory. For those of you who aren't familiar with the Unified Field Theory it deals with the existence of one overall force in the world governing all physical forces. Prior to his theory in 1925 you had five forces, (electricity, gravity, magnetism etc..) that "ran" the universe. We believe that the woman's Self-esteem is the "overall governing force" of a woman's psyche. It's "the" singular force that governs or has a dramatic effect on all her feminine feelings and actions?

Regardless of who is responsible for the loss of her self-esteem if you're attached to the woman you'll be responsible for the deficit. Daddy may have fucked her all up with inferiority complexes or whatever, but you'll be the bill payer for it's corrections, (sucks to be you).

Attacks on a female's poor self esteem can happen during childhood secondary to an abusive event, high school, date rape, violent rape, sex too early, sex too late, incest, infidelity on a man's part, infidelity in her part, poor performance in the work place, you just being a controlling asshole, body image or the fact that it's Monday, (see hormones – chapter 1). The causes and fixes are as replete as the stars in the sky. What we want you to understand is that practically any significant emotional event has the potential to attack and destroy a woman's self esteem. Get the picture?

Why is this important? If a woman's self esteem becomes severe and left untreated it can cause a myriad of problems for your relationship and of course you. As we said earlier a woman must feel worthy of happiness. Men's self esteem appears more durable than the woman's. Men tend to follow strong figures like Nietzsche, (German philosopher) who basically said that what doesn't kill you will make you stronger. They tend to feel worthy of happiness almost innately. Women on the other hand appear to have trouble and have to work at it. Low self-esteem can make a woman not feel "sexy" giving you very poor quality of sex destroying your relationship with her. Or she has such a low self esteem that she becomes a mark for other men to use her. She might be so fucked up self-esteem wise that she needs immediate gratification from sex, shopping or drugs, (or have a baby) to bring her some sort of happiness. Of course these actions will never be her fault because she's a woman and that's synonymous with victim. Remember: Postulate #1: SHE WILL FORGIVE BUT SHE WILL NEVER FORGET.

The Crypt of Memories. If the female suffers significant self esteem attacks during childhood she can and sometimes does "shelve" her self-esteem issues, (everyone has the potential to do this). If necessary she can box her bad feelings up and hide them deep in the back of her mind for years, (ex. Remember all of those repressed child molestation accusations a few years ago). Some of these were bullshit, and some were really most sincerely real. In the real ones the bad feelings came back and the damage along with them. These situations can occur when a female's life is at idle, or a similar event takes place to allow her mind the opportunity for the demons to resurface. Other events can trigger this as well.

Actions on the objective. If you have already built a life with her you now have to help her exorcise her demons. That involves helping her to resolve her issues to move on with your relationship. Note: Don't have a child to help her "fix" her self esteem issues. Having a child does help women in the short run, but eventually her issues will resurface and will have to be dealt with. This would only be more difficult if she has the stresses of parenthood to cope with. This all too common and makes you an indentured financial servant to her for many years. Mental/psyche problems typically amplify with the passage of time.

The key here is to attempt to identify these self-esteem deficits if present while dating, cohabitating or in the first three years of childless marriage. If you discover a severe deficit and you don't want to carry that cross then you should dump her completely and immediately. I know this is a tough hard core stand to make, but we don't advise what to do either way. We want you to identify the situation so you can make an informed decision.

CONSTITIUENTS OF POOR SELF ESTEEM

The following will familiarize you with some of the causes of poor self esteem.

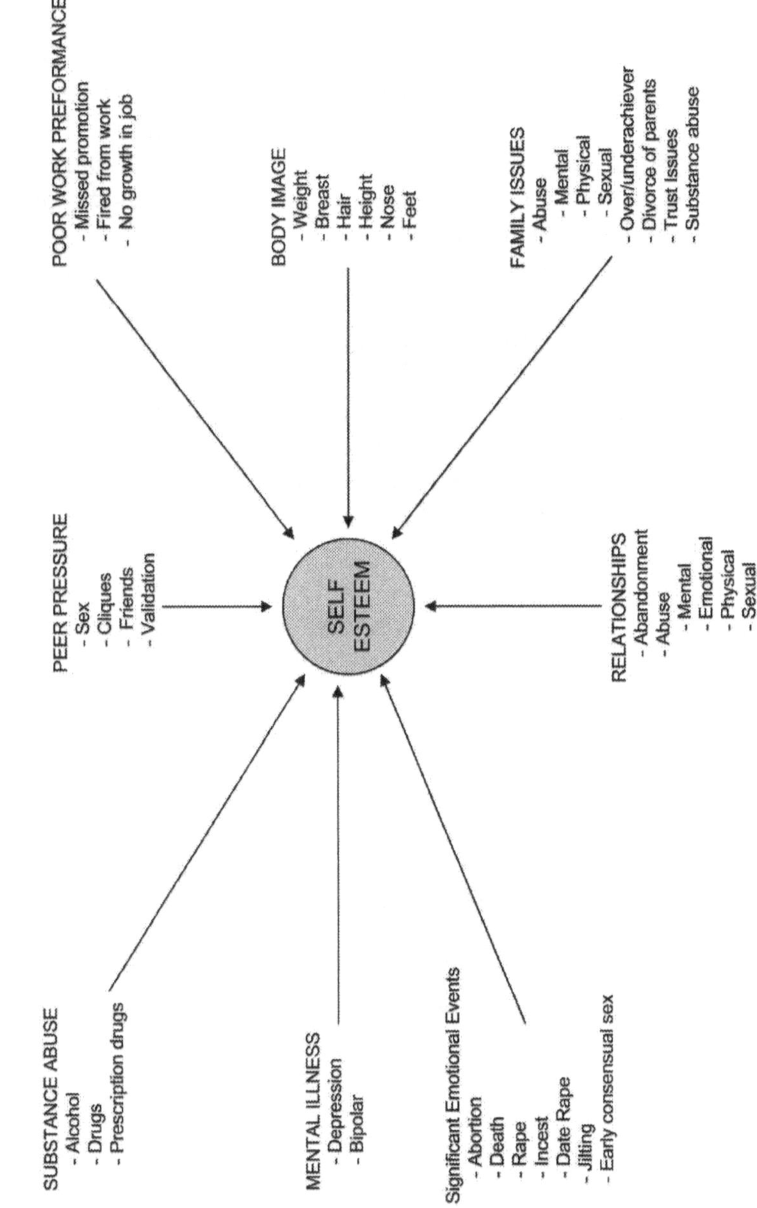

1. Body Image. We believe this is one of the earliest attacks on a woman's self esteem, (other than abuse). Today women are forced into the "Barbie image". That is big tits, little waist, nice tight ass, silky hair, peaches and cream completion and of course no fat. Men love it and women blame their inferiority on men's desires. However, if it's a man's fault, why do Vogue, Elle and all the other WOMEN'S magazines hawk this type of woman? Why don't they profile the naturally beautiful woman, (read plump)? They're in the business to sell magazines. Women buy these magazines, (not men) supporting the big titted, skinny waisted Barbies they hate. t's what women want.

   War Story. I have a lesbian friend and I occasionally hang out with her and her lesbian friends. I thought I would see women seeking or being attracted to the "inner beauty" women all men are encouraged by feminist groups to marry. This is all looks aside; use only personality and no physical attributes to determine mate selection. What I saw was that these women aren't attracted to the pleasingly plump babes with great personalities. Most of them wanted the BARBIES!

   The men love 'em but so do the women. The female is as much a victim of her own vanity as the man who desires it. So at an early age women start to be concerned about their body image. Some of these are:

   a) Weight. Most important and popular overall. Biggest detractor. Some writers indicate this is the first attack on the female self-esteem starting as early as five years old. In reality, most men will take a skinny ugly bitch over a 300-pound glob of shit that's beautiful. Insurance companies are now looking into obese people secondary to the health care cost associated with their weight. Fat people cost more for health care. Everybody is down on fat. The airlines have for years charged 2x the price for super fat passengers who can't fit into just one seat. The military and some major corporations are requiring everybody to maintain a certain weight and being overweight is counted negatively on their job reviews.

      Actions on the objective. It would be helpful for the male to examine the struggle of his girl's weight during her life. Was it hard for her to control? Was she ever fat? If she was fat does she exhibit any signs of current or past eating disorders or low self-esteem? Look for these;

they have the potential for disaster if pathological. Is body appearance a major "load bearing wall" of her self-esteem? Gaining weight later on in life will undoubtedly cost you something. Look at her mother's weight now. Most likely she'll be somewhere close to her mother's weight eventually, (this is not a rule). Also look at the girl's ankles. Thick ankles could mean big weight gain somewhere down the road.

b) Breasts. Second most popular. Most men love big tits. We don't know why, we just do. This will also include nipples, (big is always better). Shape is less important, but still in the judges corner. Sag. Large breasted women will dread the scourge of gravity and age. Big tits are great but gravity will eventually affect them sooner or later. This is especially true if she likes to "show them off" by going braless a lot. The breasts have ligaments inside called "the suspensory ligaments of Cooper". These give the breast the "perky appearance" men so much love during the female's young years. As the ravage of time and pregnancies takes its effect, the ligaments will stretch and these once lovely trophies will begin to sag. Prevention/ minimizing the damage will require the woman to wear a heavy bra most of the time, strap her self up like a Victorian woman to jog or exercise and be very careful going braless. Even this won't guarantee success but a woman will do this rather than have two eggs hanging off a nail later. Women who are used to having the attention of men admiring her mammalian protuberances, (tits) would have a potential self-esteem attack if something happens to these things, (i.e. breast cancer, stretch marks etc.)

c) Others. Nose, hair, feet, height are some of the others. Virtually any sub-standard body part is up for grabs by the woman.

Body image is a major constituent of self-esteem. Close attention should focus on the priority she places on her body image. Concern is good, obsession is bad. As time goes on her beauty will of course start to fade. If she's made her body image a major load-bearing wall of her self esteem then you could be in for some big trouble. Tit jobs for the sagging tits, tummy tucks for the belly and stretch marks, face-lifts and liposuction are just some of the options. Did I mention you would be the bill payer? Either you listen to the wailing of her lost youth or pay out the surgery fees. Oh by the way, cosmetic surgery usually isn't covered by insurance. It's 100% out of pocket. So you might not want to dump that small-breasted girl you're dating. If she doesn't get surgery or it fails then she might feel the need to pump up other areas, (build other walls) to feel good, (keep the roof up). Clothes, cars, houses, alcohol, drugs, indiscriminant sexual partners or a brand new man are some of these.

BREAST CANCER

Breast cancer effects a large population of women today. There are women who unfortunately have to undergo a "mastectomy" secondary to breast cancer. This is medical talk for removal of the breast. Just the mention of this will run fear down any woman's spine, (even ones with healthy self esteem). The insult to the self-esteem that a woman undergoes is tremendous and debilitating. Only well grounded and stable women are able to survive this operation with their self-esteem intact. If you have a female who has to undergo this operation and has many "load bearing" walls regarding her appearance, then you could be in for some problems. This is, of course, not a sign to leave her, (if you thought about this then you're a fuck stick). It's time to give her your greatest support and to seek qualified professional counseling immediately for both of you. She'll desperately need it and so will you.

2. Significant Emotional Events. Everybody has these and everybody can react differently to the same event. Anything significant that happens to a woman during her life has the potential to damage her self-esteem. We call the SEEs, (significant emotional events). Without getting "knee deep" in these, we will give a partial list of them for example:
    a. Abortion
    b. Date rape
    c. Violent rape
    d. Incest
    e. Early consensual sex
    f. Jilted by lover
    g. Homosexuality
    h. Death of parent

i. Death of a friend
j. Alienation of peers during school years
k. Etc. etc…

The list can go on and on. Remember we're trying to help you simply ID the problem. If a woman will talk about her life it's a good sign. Even if she has SEEs, she might have already dealt with them. Just because she had an abortion doesn't mean she's FUBAR, (fucked up beyond all recognition). She might have come to grips with the situation and it's not an issue for her any more. If she prefers to remain silent then you think there might be a problem.

THE POST ABORTION WOMAN

We would like to address abortion at this time. While the authors of this book personally don't condone abortion we feel that we must address its effect on women and their self-esteem.

Abortion has been around for hundreds of years but only recently has it been made legal, (Wade vs. Roe, 1973). Since that time a growing number of women have had an abortion. Which means that as time goes on the likely hood of you hooking up with a female who have had an abortion increases.

Abortion involves the death of a fetus which is a conscious decision made by the female, (and possibly influenced by her mother or boyfriend). Since the argument of when the fetus is a life is still current and very hot, women have many guilt feelings about it. Did I murder my child? These are powerful feelings they alone have to bear. And the hardest judge is themselves. Typically they bare this guilt in silence, but the conflict can be expressed in other ways. It appears that most women have a tough time reconciling their actions regardless of what they tell themselves. They'll usually carry this burden through out their lives. Knowingly or unknowingly you might get to help carry it as well.

War Story. My second wife had admitted to me that she had an abortion while a junior in high school, (influenced by her mother). I found out about this after we were married. Other than a rare tearful moment, she refused to ever talk about it and it was sudden death if I ever pursued it. Even the mention of it on television made her tearful. I don't believe that to this day she ever got over her actions and never will. She had low self esteem, and was a "never truly happy" woman. I believe that the abortion, and her guilt , prevented her from achieving true happiness, (they're other factors but this was one of the larger bricks in the wall).

For our purposes women who have had an abortion should be scrutinized, (but shouldn't have a scarlet letter stuck on them). The potential for self-esteem damage is great with a woman who has had an abortion. It's a good sign is if the woman will talk about it. If a woman can freely talk about her abortion easily she has probably reconciled it in her mind and her God. Whether it is right or wrong, it's her reaction to the abortion that is most important. Conversely if she tells you it's her choice of birth control and she's had eight of them you might want to think that one over real hard.

3. Family issues. This is a large category and can encompass anything relating to the family.
    a. Abuse. Mental, physical or sexual. Any of these can do a number on the woman. They typically happen early on and are very hard to detect and correct. Watch the family interactions or over compensating by the female.
    b. Divorce of parents. Important for the early date investigations. Since the divorce rate is approximately 50%, the likely hood of one (or both) of you will have parents that are divorced. Some questions to ask are: What age was she when her parents divorced? What's her current concept of marriage? Stepfathers? How many? Relationship with them? Were they abusive? Did her Daddy abandon her after the divorce? Current relationship with her Daddy. If Daddy directly or indirectly fucked her up this could easily lead into trust issues, inferiority issues or depression. Does she look at you as Daddy, (We know that this is fucked up, but it does happen sometimes)? They say little girls marry their fathers.
    c. Lack of attention. A situation where lack of or perceived lack of support/approval results in damaged self esteem (normally when considering the period of youth and the effects of the parental impact). Some girls didn't get enough of Daddy's attention and they have their bloomers in a knot.
    d. Substance abuse of parents. Did Mommy or Daddy have a "problem"? Substance abuse is thought to be genetic. So even if she escapes it, your children might not. Although not a showstopper, it's an area of concern.
4. Relationships. How many relationships has she had? What effect had they had on her.

   a. Multiple relationships. How many relationships did she have prior to you? How long did they last? If possible to know why did they not work out? These are all questions that can point to emotionally damaged women.
   b. Abusive. Did any of her past men beat her? Sexually abuse her? Was emotionally abusive to her? Abusive relationships with men can indicate major self-esteem issues.
   c. Abandonment. Does she have a history of men abandoning her? Even though you're a nice guy, she might have severely damaged self-esteem because she has dated guys who leave her all of the time. Is she a "storm damaged boat", (see chapter 6, finding the mate)? Is she looking for a nice man harbor to make repairs in?

5. Mentally unstable. Some women have a true "chemical in-balance" that prevents them from achieving and maintaining a minimal level of happiness. It has to do with the level of neuro-transmitters in the brain. They can lead to depression and eventually "self medication". Self-medication usually takes the form of alcohol or drugs. When this happens the woman eventually spirals into some self-esteem shattering events, (sexual depravation, abusive relationships etc.) Some are controlled or in the early undiagnosed stages of instability, (see chapter 6, finding the mate).
6. Substance Abuse. This has warning signs all around it. We believe when a woman has a substance abuse issue it's potential indicator of an underlying problem. A few drinks, a joint here and there is acceptable for our purposes. Black out drunk, frequently drunk or stoned or drinking every night is a problem. She doesn't wish to deal with her problems, she wants to escape from her unhappiness for awhile. Alcohol will anesthetize the problem. Take away the pain and I can be happy at least for a while.
7. Peer Pressure. Young females are constantly pelted with pressures from peers. Earliest assaults can be "cliques". The group she "hangs out with". Which group, what's their social standing with in the masses. People who don't have a group face social isolation, ridicule and no validation. This of course extends to what the group thinks of sex. Is it cool? Etc... Then the female is faced with the young dating ritual, pressure from first loves for initial sex, demands for time. Friends play a very important part in the development of healthy self-esteem. The lack of a clique is undesirable, but the total lack of friends is disastrous. Females

without a good friend base faces extreme isolation, introverted behavior and inability to integrate into society. Reevaluate your decision on you mate if she has a poor history of friends.

This is only some of the potential constitinuents of poor self-esteem. We listed some of the larger obvious ones for an example. It's a lot to understand, but it's so important for a woman to have a good self-esteem. She has to be on top of her game to be on top of you.

EFFECTS OF POOR SELF ESTEEM

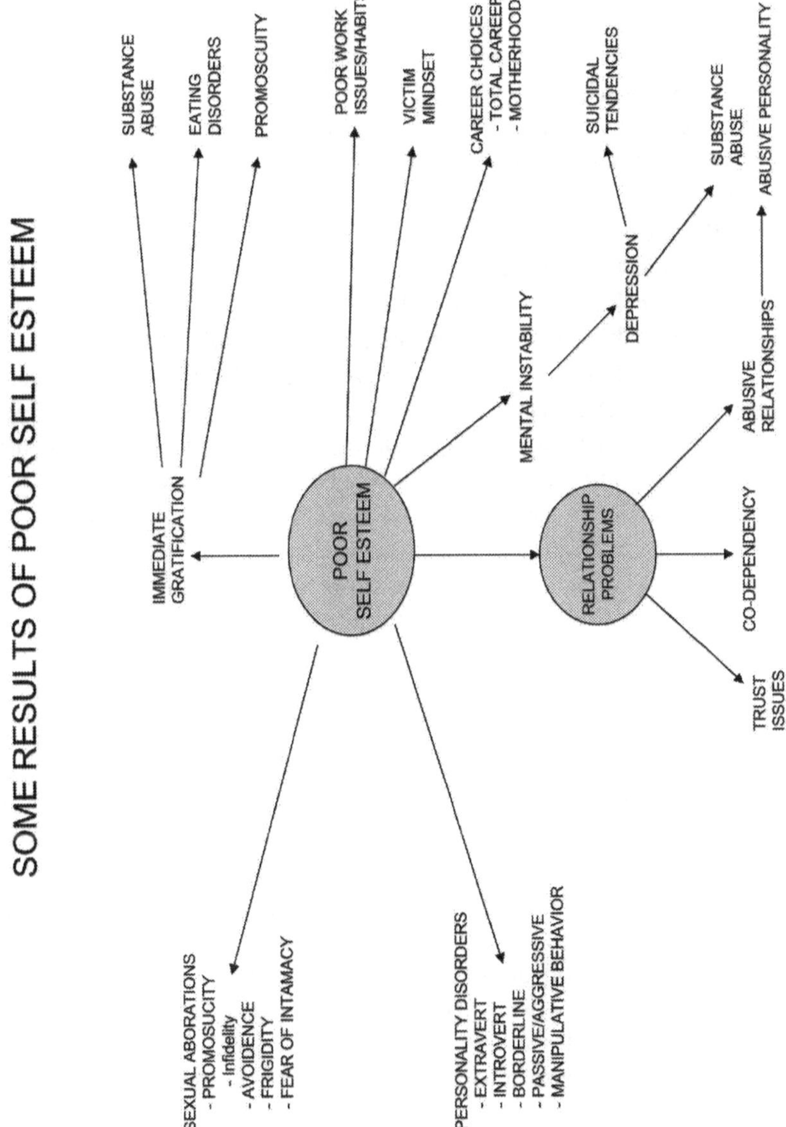

The causes of low self-esteem are subtle. If you have trouble recognizing some of these potential causes, you might recognize some of the symptoms or results of low self-esteem. When we observe a woman in abnormal actions the average guy simply writes it off to being a girl or whatever. He hasn't a clue why she acted the way she did and many times he probably doesn't care. But to a woman who has a near-pathological or pathological self esteem deprivation her actions sometimes can be identified. This identification can save your life, (and your wallet).

1. Relationship Issues. When women have suffered a loss of self-esteem, they can express it in many ways. Especially in their relationships with men. Many times relationship issues invade relationships and can be manifested in the following:
    a. Trust. One of the key ingredients of a successful relationship is the ability to trust the other mate. Lack of trust plagues many couples. It can be displayed in security issues and jealously. This deficiency can fester and grow into a large entity that engulfs the couple for minor issues. Without the ability for the woman to trust her mate the probability of successful relations is poor. Her insecurity can cause the male to spend an enormous amount of time and energy to reassure the woman that her lack of trust is unfounded. That he's a good guy bullshit, bullshit, bullshit.....

       War Story. Gerald and Dee had been dating for almost five years. This in itself has caused some insecurity issues with Dee who already had a steamer trunk of self-esteem issues from prior relationships. Gerald had been married/ divorced and has his own baggage regarding marriage. But now he has decided to "up" the status of their relationship by allowing Dee to move in, (which is what she has wanted). The move was accomplished but since the "honeymoon" has turned disastrous. Dee is always accusing him of being unfaithful. But Dee's insecure actions are actually poisoning the cohabitation. Each day she checks his cell phone, house phone and his wallet for artifacts of infidelity. This causes Gerald to constantly spend time and emotional energy to reassure her that he isn't cheating on her. Her paranoia has continued so long he is now considering having her move out.
    b. Codependency. This is another relationship issue. Because of a large lack of self-esteem the woman becomes

so dependent on the man she is "codependent" on him for her emotional survival. Codependency is one of those 100,000-book subject we won't get into. If you think she's too dependent on you, then you must read on your own or seek professional help. If she displays some of the following characteristics then you might want to do some research.

1) My good feelings about who I am stem from being liked by you.
2) My good feelings about who I am stem from receiving approval from you.
3) My mental attention is focused on you.
4) My mental attention is focused on manipulating you to do it my way.
5) My own hobbies/interests are put aside. My time is spent sharing your hobbies and interests.
6) I am not aware of how I feel, I am aware of how you feel.
7) My fear of rejection determines what I say or do.
8) My fear of your anger determines what I say or do.
9) I put my values aside in order to connect with you.
10) The quality of my life is in relation to the quality of yours.

If you see some of these characteristics then you want to look deeper into your prospective mate. Seek professional help. These type of behaviors lead to a dead end street with all of your energy consumed for nothing.

<<<<<<< WARNING WARNING>>>>>>>>

c. Abusive relationships. If the woman demonstrates abuse to you or to others this is a serious warning sign. Abusive relationships are usually a learned behavior. It can be a stand-alone action or the vanguard to much deeper issues. If physical abuse is experienced early on in the relationship then terminate the relationship immediately. Physical abuse to you could be physical abuse to your children. This should be a no brainer Einstien. There's no excuse for physical abuse.

2. Sexual issues. As we said earlier, when one load bearing wall is missing another is usually established to prevent a collapse. When a woman has severe self-esteem deficiency, it can be expressed in many ways. One of the ways the female seeks immediate gratification is through sexual outlets. Little quick and easy joys provide the necessary boosts to the self-esteem. This has its own self-fulfilling prophecy though.
   Example. A female has a shitty fucked up childhood. Her self-esteem is low secondary to poor finances, poor role models and no spiritual guidance for values or some abusive event(s). She finds out relatively early that leading the pack in sex places her in a much more celebrated position then she was previously. She has the attention of many boys, maybe entrance into a clique and some validation. However this sexual promiscuity doesn't solve her dilemma, it just pays the interest on her problems. Eventually the debt will have to be paid. Her sexually sponsored popularity will soon die off when other girls eventually "ante up" to the sexual dating pot. She could raise the stakes by raising her sexual participation or kinky-ness. But eventually she'll generally "level out" with her peers or age will catch up with her. When that happens she'll be faced with her initial problems to solve (and probably some extra ones as well).

IMMEDIATE GRATIFICATION

In America live in an age of instancy. This is a byproduct of the industrial world in which we live. We are all bombarded by the ever-increasing need to respond to the technological demands of our "instant" society. We have been in a deluge of "instants". Fast food, fast oil changes, and finally fast relationships. Technology and our industrial capacity has erased the need to fix things because it is cheaper and faster to trash it and buy new ones, so it appears to be the same with relationships.

Women by their nature tend to live in the immediate gratification zone. A good book to learn about this is "The Tender Warrior". The author accurately describes the God given roles about men and women. He lists an analogy of a wagon train heading west. We as men are like the scout, searching for today's campsite, but thinking 2-3 campsites/days down the road. The woman who is in the wagon is consumed not with the choice of campsite today or tomorrow, she's worried about the here and now. Are the children warm, safe? Will we have water? Do we have food for the evening meal? If he doesn't get some game to eat tonight what will I Fix to eat?

You see, it's in a woman's nature to focus on the immediate. The man's nature is typically about the future. God made it this way for a purpose. He placed man in charge because he sees the forest, while the woman sees the trees. Both of these views are important for survival. Which make both views necessary for a successful relationship. Eliminating one view would leave the family unit incomplete and it would eventually flounder and disintegrate. Together they not only survive but they thrive.

What the man needs to know is that though immediate gratification is necessary for some occasions many times there's a price to be paid. Excessive concern about immediate gratification is a sign of poor self-esteem. They need to have many little "joys" at the expense of a delayed joy. This can lead to poor planning, poor confidence in one's ability and generally shallow thinking. Watch your Mrs. Candidate closely if she has trouble with excessive immediate gratification. This is especially important if one of her immediate things happens to be sex. Healthy individuals understand delayed gratification.

Women's immediate gratification was held in check by the potential of pregnancy. This was a brake that slowed the fright train of pleasure down to a manageable speed. Now with the advent of birth control and abortion women have virtually nothing holding them back in the pursuit of their immediate happiness. Beware of the immediate gratification that exceeds the normal variant that accompanies the average woman. If immediate gratification urges are excessive then investigate potential pathological issues within the self-esteem of your mate.

DENIAL

This is an important topic to be discussed regarding women. Denial is simply where a person either consciously or unconsciously perceives something other than the facts of any given situation. Men can live in denial but women have a very strong tendency to operate in "denial" mode. This mental state can also be a defense mechanism as well as a desired operating system. Women of all incomes, background and cultures appear to do this well. Denial can be lived out for years even when confronted, may not believe the truth.

War Story. Jean had gotten married right out of college. She was from a good family, but had never had a job secondary to her own family's needs. Unfortunately Jean was married to Kevin (who was a fuck stick). He repeatedly whored around on her and couldn't care less about the kids.

On occasionally would go out with them on the weekends. But his favorite saying was "I work all week I need this time to relax". Jean had several friends that would confront her over the years regarding her husbands whoring ways. Jean would brush it off saying it was only a "business lunch" or something like that. Eventually reality set in when Kevin fucked some whore at work and got her knocked up. They divorced and Jean eventually got on with her life. When you talked to her she wasn't so angry about his actions as she was hers. She realized that she lived in this false reality for eleven years. She was mostly mad about her "pretending" and all of the time she wasted on Kevin.

This is only one of the many forms that denial can be in. Denial isn't limited to relationships. People can live out their personal lives in denial as well. The alcoholic, the drug abuser and even the whore who thinks she's a nice girl. Anyone can lie in denial. People in denial can give creditable performances for their alternate realities. First they BELIEVE in it themselves. Second they typically have perfected their self "lie" over time so it's well practiced.

Actions on the objective. Because it's difficult to quickly determine a pathological denial, time is our friend here. Given enough time the man can examine the woman and eventually she won't be able to substantiate her claims. So take your time and observe your woman. If she rushes you then step back and observe even longer.

BASIC NEEDS OF WOMEN

Women have some basic needs, (so do men but this book isn't about us). First let's look at everyone's basic needs. Some of you might have heard of it. It's called "Maslow's Hierarchy of Needs". It starts with the most basic of needs and continues down the list. The are:

1) Air. Need it period.
2) Water. Can last seven days until death. Need it eventually.
3) Food. Can last 30 -40 days until death. Need it eventually.
4) Shelter. Dependent on environment. Need it eventually.
5) Clothes. Dependent on environment. Need it eventually
6) Knicks season tickets. Need it period.
7) Companionship. Dependent on personality. Maybe need it.
8) Love. Dependent on personality. Maybe need it.
9) Fulfillment. Dependent on personality. Maybe need it.

This is a partial list and can be argued on some points. Items 1-6 that's pretty much a given. Items 7-9 are open to debate for priority and order. There are many more items that can be listed. But the concept here is that we all have a list of what we need to survive. Some are concrete non-negotiable items. Others are open to interpretation and compromise. Your job is to decipher what the list is for your mate and after negotiation, attempt to fulfill them.

Dr. Harley, a Massachusetts psychologist, states that there are five basic needs for men and women. For women they are:

1) Affection
2) Communication
3) Openness and honesty
4) Financial support
5) Family commitment

Now this list isn't "cut in stone". It is right for some and might need modification for others. It doesn't even include the first five of Maslow's, (but that's pretty much a given). What key here is that a list does in fact exists. Maybe not on a conscious level, but it does exists. This is a good "starting point".

For reference the list Dr. Harley gives for men is as follows:

1) Sexual fulfillment, (big fucking surprise right?)
2) Recreational companionship, (let's go fishing)
3) An attractive wife
4) Domestic support
5) Admiration

What we have here are two completely different schools of thought. It's amazing that we even get together long enough to procreate. But we thank God we do. Keep this list in mind when you try to "logically" decipher your mate out. What makes sense to you using your value system won't work here. The list above is an example of a list, but everyone is different. So it's going to be pretty much a trial and error event.

ALL IN ALL

We believe that the core of a woman's actions, feelings, and emotions stem from her self-esteem. You must always be aware that there are a myriad of destructive forces pummeling the females self-esteem throughout her life. If you recognize a "pathological" or severe loss of your female's self-esteem then you have the knowledge to act. You may "tuff it out" or bail depending on how young the relationship is, if you're married or have children or how you feel about her. This is your choice not ours. We show you what we have encountered.

CHAPTER 4

THE DIGITAL-ANALOG MALE-FEMALE INTERFACE

What we are going to talk about is another CORNERSTONE concept. Earlier we talked about the female's self esteem and how it governs her emotional world. We also talked about how the man thinks and the woman feels, the need for a woman to have discussion with someone during her day and the man's response to that. Now we're going to talk about how the female views her ideas of her world and how the male views his ideas. This is important because we believe that the man processes, categorizes and stores information differently than the female. His is an active conscious process and we believe that hers is a more passive unconscious effort. He thinks he hears what she is at that time. She thinks he heard it. But for some reason he screws it up, (her thoughts) and he thinks she's just a crazy bitch and doesn't know what she wants. Have we ever been here before?

There's a myriad of books out there trying to help men listen, understand and talk to a woman. Most men really want to please a woman. We know that old equation PLEASURE OF THE WOMAN = PLEASURE OF THE MAN. Men keep looking for that special instruction book. You know that book that we can look up a situation in it, follow the emotional recipe and all will be right with the world. By now men are beginning to find out that the holy grail of books doesn't exist. So the only thing men are left to do is listen. They can pretend we're from Mars and she's from Venus to try and talk blah, blah, blah. Don't get me wrong; it's a great book and recommend it's reading. The thing that men have to do is realize that women process external facts, emotions and feelings differently then men. A simile would be like we have two different computer operating systems. The output is the same but one system can't talk to the other system. Suffice to say men are "digital" and women are "analog". We could say, "Men are from IBM and Women are from Apple".

DIGITAL PACKAGING

Let's say that men do think in a digital sense. We take our important ideas, emotions and feelings and package them in nice little mental "packets". We line them up and once we have all of the items we want we prioritize them for importance, pleasure or criticality, (see diagram below). This little "flow chart" is the picture of the male's mental process. Simple is best… less is more that's how men like it. Life is good in their world because it's neat, orderly and CONSISTANT. It makes perfect sense to them and allows them to tackle any problems that may arise by stating the following problem solving "mantra";

1) Analyze the problem
2) Make a plan
3) Execute the plan
4) Supervise the plan
5) Evaluate the plan.

Men love this mantra and use it at every opportunity, (it's in their "nature"). Once complete we put it in their little logical model, they package it, prioritize it, schedule the solution, conquer it and life goes on.

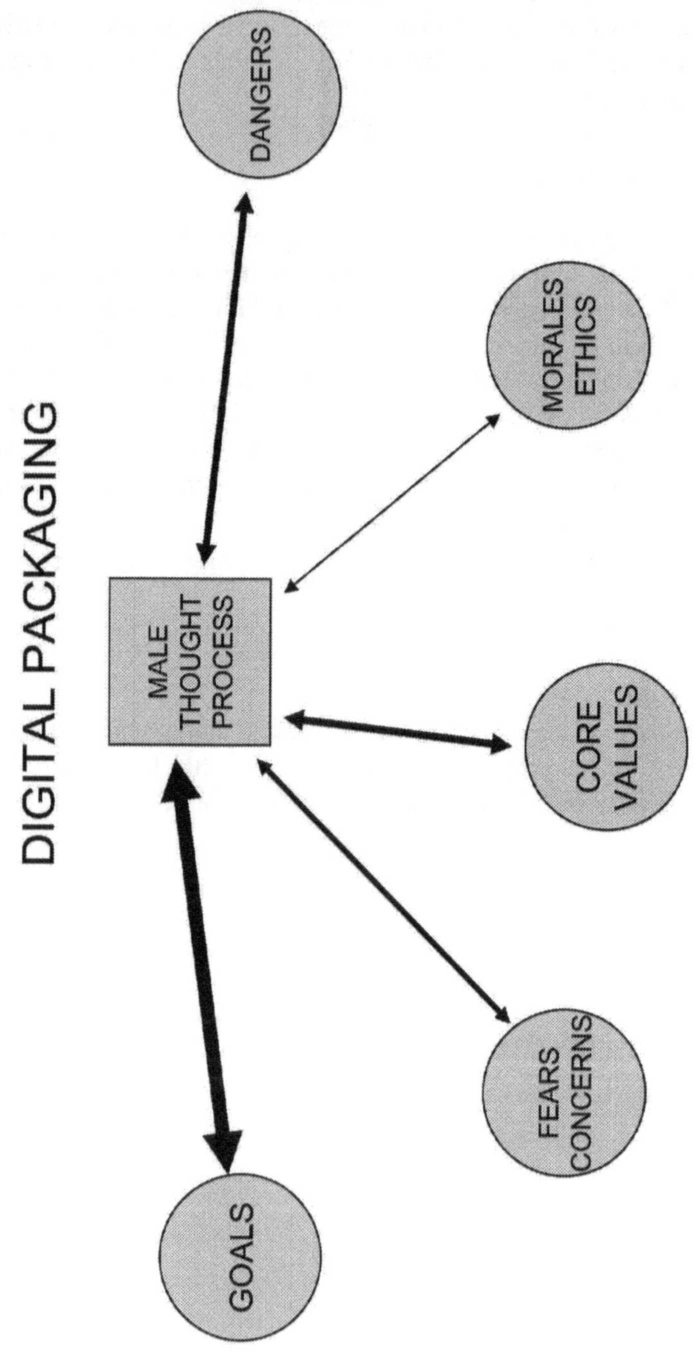
DIGITAL PACKAGING
MALE THOUGHT PROCESS
DANGERS
MORALES ETHICS
CORE VALUES
FEARS CONCERNS
GOALS

ANALOG PACKAGING

Now let's look at the analog world of the female. We've talked about an experiment in the Book "Brain Sex" that documents the equality that exists in men and women's mental capacity. It also proves that even though men and women have the same answers the solutions they're processed in different areas of the brain. Looking at the diagram below we see the representation of the female's mental process looking very much like a river. One thing to keep in mind, rivers by definition isn't static, (if they were they'd be pond water). They FLOW carrying all sorts of shit down stream. This is similar to the woman; she has HER emotions, goals, ideas and feelings the same as men do. But the difference is that the woman's packets aren't set up in a static environment that allow for a good orderly formation. They're kind of like "plankton", (this is the very small sea life that whales eat, they have no propulsion and depend entirely upon outside forces to move). Since there packets aren't fixed in place like the man's they can, (and usually do), move up and down the mental river in varying positions. Like the plankton, they kind of flow according to the obstacles (rocks, bends and banks) of the river. These obstacles we see in her "river" are usually significant emotional events, (a man, biological time clock, death, work etc…). There is no real prioritizing done here it's totally dependent upon the ever changing outside environment. Note: Women can through their "male side" adopt the static model. But it doesn't usually stay in the male static mode forever. Eventually the river will start to flow.

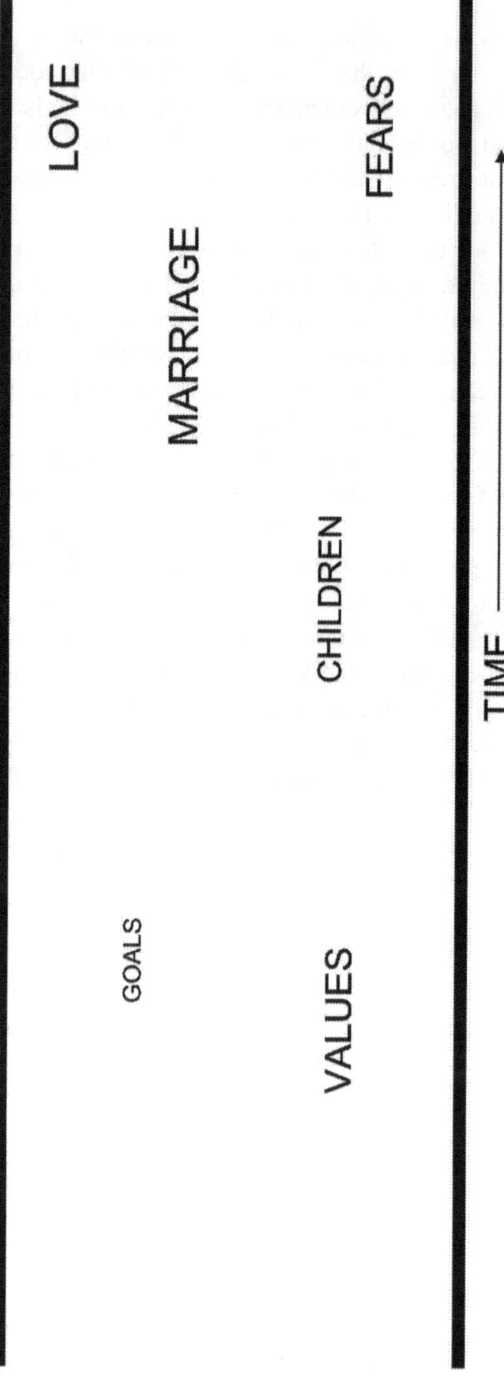
ANALOG PACKAGING
GOALS
VALUES
CHILDREN
MARRIAGE
LOVE
FEARS
TIME

THE DIGITAL ANALOG INTERFACE

Here's where the fun begins. When men and women "get together" they typically want to connect. Men typically like to do this physically, (sex) and women usually do this emotionally, (talking about feelings and shit). The woman particularly needs this connection to operate effectively. The man… well it's okay too, but not needed nearly as much as the woman needs it. Where problems arise is when the man looks at his woman. He takes mental a "snapshot" of her at that particular moment. Now armed with this mental blueprint of his woman's mental make-up, he immediately processes the information packets, aligns them, stores them, prioritizes them, saving them for any potential problems.

If a problem arises, he simply pulls out his mental blueprint, chants the mantra and takes action on whatever he sees is the problem for his mate. Is he wrong? No, but he's a little short on being right. The man didn't realize that once he got the snapshot of her "state" the situation had already started to morph, (and the river continues to flow). As we look at the diagram below we see that the snap shot the man had taken shows one static picture. This is different than the earlier diagram isn't it? That's because the mental river has flowed and those concepts that were important no longer have the same precedence as they previously did. What may have been a perfect solution for an issue or problem was now based on old intelligence and no longer a valid plan. Her make-up had changed and it was leaving him desperately behind the power-curve. What does he do now? Well it's back to his tried and true problem solving techniques. He chants his mantra, pulls out his snapshot of his woman, makes a plan, initiates it and all the other good stuff only realizing that he's missing the point again, (and It was a damn good plan). Now with some frustration he gets caught in a loop-back that he goes over and over because he knows that by using this process he will eventually stumble on the right solution. The female becomes frustrated because he just doesn't GET IT! Now with frustration and anxiety they start to…. fight. With both of them vying to get their point across because they know their way works.

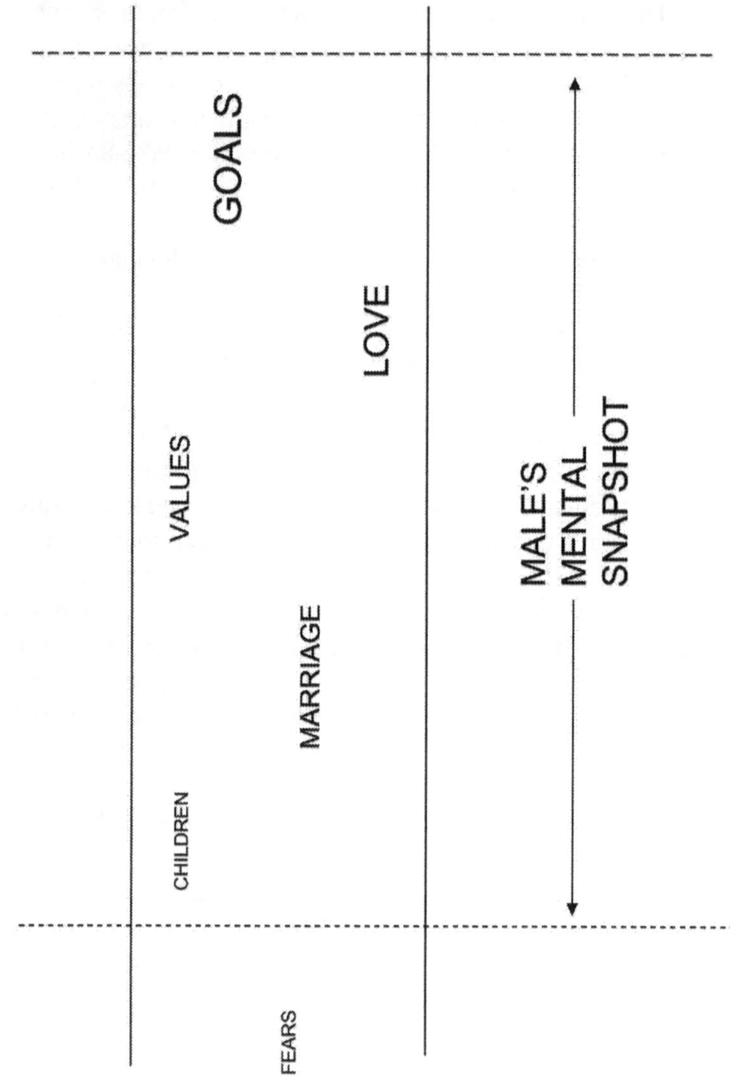
DIGITAL-ANALOG INTERFACING
GOALS
VALUES
CHILDREN
LOVE
MARRIAGE
FEARS
MALE'S
MENTAL
SNAPSHOT

In his mental snapshot he didn't even see her "fears". That was left out of the whole picture. But earlier it was at the forefront of the earlier picture. Later on when the "river flows" her "fears" may go to the front of her "scope" and he's left with the question "What the fuck happened? She didn't have any fears when I met her"?

To make things even more interesting… We have noticed that the river doesn't flow at the same rate. The "current" may be slow, or at times speeds up. Some women have chronically high "currents" which can be commensurate to "shooting the rapids". A lot of fun sure, but is this the way you want to live ALL of you life? The choice is yours.

War Story. Greg met Sharon in their third year of college. Sharon was exactly like Greg exciting, driven and very goal oriented. After three years they had become engaged and she had moved in. Greg was in graduate school for art and Sharon was finishing her MBA. When they were done they had planned several years of working overseas. After a while Sharon had expressed much doubt about working overseas. She had said the pay wasn't that good, it could be dangerous and it would hamper them getting their "start" in their professions. Greg looked at the problem and applied his problem solving mantra. He took each question she had and solved it to his satisfaction, (unfortunately not to her satisfaction). What had happened was that Greg had been using his old mental snap shot of Sharon. She had, during that time of school and fun, her river flow and now she had, because of her biological time clock, caused the packet "children" to "flow" to the front of her priorities. Now she didn't want to work over seas and "see the world". She had "baby-itits", and wanted to establish herself at work and start a family. Greg, after many long discussions and arguments, figured out what Sharon really wanted. He made the decision to stay in the US and allow Sharon to start work. They eventually started a family.

Actions on the objective. The man needs to be aware of the difference in the operating system of the female. He needs to tailor his plans to accommodate her ever-changing environment. Not an easy task because he must make his plan very dynamic. He should ask himself two questions prior to settling down with a particular female:

1) How fast is her current? Look at the amount of drama in her life and try to determine how much of it is internally generated. If she "falls on her own sword" frequently step back and look her over from a distance. Fast current women will always have a lot of drama in their life. You could be forced to "shoot the rapids" for many issues. Remember: Slow current = more stability but

if you get too slow of a river it could be boring. You need some current/movement. Always seek moderation.

2) How many bends/obstacles are in her emotional river? Again try to "map" out her river. Rocks/bends = old issues, new issues, childhood, significant emotional events or pathological manifestations of self esteem. These in turn can move her priorities ahead faster or slow them down. Rivers typically are never straight forever.

Before he attempts to solve a problem he has to assess her mental priority status. What does the snap shot look like right now? The female isn't wrong and neither is the man. They're just two different operating systems and the man must be the integrator.

CHAPTER 5

THE ROLE OF THE WOMAN IN THE NEW WORLD ORDER

So far in this book we have painted a grim picture of women. We only want to detail the "undesirable female",(they're good ones out there). We want to outline what we call for our purposes "pathological". These are the ones we want you to watch out for. We don't advocate women hooking up with "undesirable men", (fuck sticks) either. Now want to describe what the "old world" female, (Mom) was like and what her stresses were like. Then add the female of today and the new stresses/challenges that she has to deal with in this new world order, (NWO).

MOM AND APPLE PIE

Women in the old days had markedly fewer issues to deal with than their counterparts of the NWO. In the old days women were concerned with locating, attracting and committing to a mate, (and getting him to commit). This was for love, procreation and security. During the years of marriage the following responsibilities were theirs:

1. Wife. She was the companion found through dating to have like interests and values. A union was formed and they could pretty much count on living their life together. Her primary focus is the man.
2. Nest builder. Her job was to assemble the nest, (home) and keep it in a functioning status, (housework). Additional duties were to

care for the husband and children, (food, nurturing the children and husband. Her primary focus is still the man, but is preparing for her offspring.

3. Mother. To have offspring, raise them primarily until school when they became the worries of the state school system. Just joking... maybe. She was the primary caretaker of the children for the first five years. This is important because the personality of a child is said to be established during this time period. Shared focus is the children and the man.

We could assemble more items on the list but for our purposes this will suffice. These were, as we see it, the "big three" areas of the Old World Woman.

A COMMUNITY OF SISTERS

If you look back to the older days you would find that the America was quite different. Men worked outside of the home and women worked inside the home. The majority of America functioned this way in sort of a functional sexual segregation. During this time when a woman encountered stress, a problem, concerns or questions she had a whole community, (neighborhood of wives/sisters) to talk out her feelings or get answers from. They would sit around their "coffee clutches" and "listen to each others problems". Of course they wouldn't get any solutions, (but then again they weren't looking for any). In this semi-communal atmosphere they would get the help they really needed. Which was somebody to tell them it was going to be all right, everything would work itself out, squirt a few tears and maybe a hug blah, blah, blah... At the end of the neighborhood therapy session they'd feel better and be able to return to their homes to carry on with their lives.

A WOMAN IN THE NEW WORLD ORDER

Nowadays women not only have the previous responsibilities that we listed above, but they have saddled themselves with traditional male roles, duties and new female challenges to contend with.

1. Employee. She must go to work and earn a wage. As we discussed earlier since WWII women have been working in increasing numbers each year. The majority of us now live within a two paycheck society. So women basically HAVE to work. Now there are couples who still live on one paycheck. We consider them exceptions and not the rule for our purposes. Since most

couples work because they have to the woman is forced to work along with the man in order for the family unit not only to survive, but to thrive.

2. Peer. This sounds strange but it's true. The stresses placed on women by their peers are enormous. In the old days pressure was in the form of their wifely duties. Good cook, clean home and nice children were the benchmarks then. The pressure supported their role. Now the peer pressure isn't just for the homemakers. It's the female media that bombards the new world woman with the reminders of "Did I waste my life by forgoing the career that I could have had"? The soap operas that paints a picture of the glamorous female executive making decisions and shaking the world up. Yes and oh by the way has a bevy of great looking men kissing her ass all the time. If she does follow this path she'll have the question "Did I waste my life ignoring my family for a career? No one lies on their death bed and wishes that they had spent more time at the office. This and many other questions lead the female to her current cognitive dissonance.
3. Job dominance. Now that we have two people working it's not as simple as it was in earlier times. Along with the stress the woman of today has to think what happens to my job if he's transferred? What happens to his job if "I'm" transferred? Whose career will have priority? This has probably been the seed crystal for many arguments these days. More stress to think about.
4. Social isolation. Even if the woman makes a conscious decision to stay home for the sake of her family, she faces a potential social isolation since the majority of women do in fact work. This voluntary confinement can drive the best women into a "crazy bitch" mode over time.

HONEY I'M HOME.......

We are detailing this to give the man a look at the stress the NWO woman has to deal with. Dr. John Grey in one of his "Men are from Mars women are from Venus" books talks about the how the man should sit back and allow the woman upon return form work to switch over to her feminine side. That she has been at work all day using her "male" side and it takes a little time for her to "morph" into the softer female side. This kind of sounds like the "Hulk", but it serves a point. In the old days the woman would stay in her feminine world exclusively and wait for the man to come home. Once home they would do the family thing. Now if the woman is to get along with the man she has to "change" sex personalities on a daily basis. What if she doesn't change fast enough? What if she doesn't want to change preferring to remain in her "man" image? (I like being IN CONTROL). Do you see the potential conflict that just this issue can cause? Or could you perhaps see the identity crisis that's percolating here?

THE GUY AT WORK

Along with ALL the other shit women have to contend with, the working woman must endure the "Guy at work". We feel this is important because a good woman if left poorly managed will turn "farrow", (return to the wild for you dummies). When a good woman is married or coupled to an idiot, (defined as someone who hasn't bought our book), and becomes neglected and abused, is an obvious mark for a hostile takeover. The woman's partner has the home team advantage but the "other guy" has the power of the "new", "different" and promising. Here's why:

1) Different doesn't mean better. Especially true for men and affects women as well. Different means… different. Even though it's not better the different has a mysterious quality to it. An allure that can't be countered. You're the same, (with all your neglect) and HE"S different, new and exciting.
2) Always nice. The other guy is always nice, he never yells, says "fuck you" or "you cunt" at the office. He's usually always in a good mood, tries to get along with people and is generally helpful. This guy sounds a lot like you are at work. See the pattern?
3) Always dressed well. The other guy is always dressed well, clean and you never see "him" on the toilet stinking up the bathroom or scratching his nuts in front of the TV.
4) The other guy always is paying her compliments. Oh you've changed you hair. I really like the new dress bullshit, bullshit, bullshit…..

These are typically things that people do at work to get along. Compliments, dressing nice and being cheerful. You do it, we do it and everybody does it. It's called being kind, courteous and congenial in the workplace. Where people get into trouble is when they meet at work and the home front isn't solid. When men and women work together the possibility exists that they can develop a romantic relationship, (yes when you put a boy hamster and a girl hamster in a cage don't bitch about the little hamsters that follow). It's the human element and anything is possible, but what are the probabilities?

Actions on the objective. Read our book. Read all the books we tell you to read. Get familure with her needs and feelings. Remember unmet demand is your "true enemy". You can reduce the probabilities by maintaining a solid bond with your mate. Good communication, understanding of all her girl shit, and sharing of the traditional duties so she doesn't feel like she's in it all alone. You're the leader, so you initiate it, (don't let her bring this to you, you bring it to her). Tell her that since she's working as well it's only fair that each partner do a share of the house work and other traditional wife duties. She will appreciate it and laud you later in the sack. It will also set the precedence that "since you're working outside the home" meaning if she ever quits all bets are off. The house work IS her job by traditional definition. These actions will keep her stable; relatively happy and satisfied she could never get such a participative partner ever, (so she better not do anything to fuck this up). If she ever did cheat on you, she would probably do so regardless of how good you were. Your only choice in our opinion is to dump her, (weigh the child support first).

MR HELPER

What does the NWO woman do when she has a problem? In the current situation she is no longer with her "sisters" all day. Does that mean that her need to talk things out is gone? No ass-wipe! She's probably unable to talk out her frustrations with her peers because the "community" she once had is now gone. Actually her "sisters" were at work where she was all day long. When these women get home they're occupied with their own families and problems to deal with. They have no time to "talk things out with the other women". So they end up talking to the only adult they can find. That's right their husbands and when they tell them their problems the men become "Mr. Helper and want to fix shit. This of course is the wrong fucking answer! So the men are in the shit soup and the women are of course victims because the men don't understand their feelings and so forth and so forth…

Actions on the Objective. Read "Men are from Mars, Women are from Venus". It's a great book that accurately describes the need for the action-less help that women desperately need. Read it regardless of your feelings about it. It's necessary mandatory reading.

In retrospect men are "action figures". No asshole, we're not GI Joe. We're creatures of action, decisive and quick is our terrible swift sword. The thought of simply providing comfort to a woman and do nothing else to solve her problem is completely foreign to us. Matter of fact it's mentally upsetting to us, (it's like taking a dump and not finishing the paperwork). It especially itches if we have a sure fire plan that we know in our hearts will work. Become accustomed with keeping your "Mr. Helper" hat off. If you want this to work out you must give her the help SHE wants. When you ask her to hold a beam so you can saw it, do you want her to ask you "How do you feel about that beam?" Or "Why do you want to nail that beam?" No you want her to hold the fucking beam. Get the picture? She's come to you for comfort, (not the shell answer man dummy) you have to give her comfort, bite your tongue, and swallow it if you have to but you do the following:

1) Let her talk. She has to clear the air, and look at the problem.
2) Hold her and reassure her that it's all going to be all right, (also make stupid soothing noises).
3) Rub her back, arms and other non-sensuous body parts. This can be really good for her to relax. DO NOT TRY TO HAVE SEX, (unless she initiates it). We know that this is always a good thing for us. But she has the problem. She might want the distraction, but she decides (the sex will come eventually and it's usually pretty good).
4) Listen to her cry or whatever shit she needs. Just the act of touch, sympathy or holding will start the waterworks. You didn't do anything wrong. She just needs to cry it out. It's the emotional release she needs. The crying resets some sort of emotional circuit breaker in her head.

The results will be obvious you special sensitive guy! Episodes like this will bond you two together, (no joking). This is especially important for other reasons, (like keeping the other guy away). If you give her what she wants, you'll get what you want eventually. Always remember "Unmet demand is your true enemy". There's always a fuck-stick out there that will be more than willing to hold her and listen to her shit, (oh yeah and fuck her too).

This is what the male has to maneuver through in the NWO. It's not like Mom and Dad had to deal with. In their day it was them against the world, survival of the family was the issue, (not their identities). They were a ship on an ocean, and all efforts were for the benefit of the ship getting to port. Now it's a whole new game and the rules are changing almost daily.

When you look at these challenges it's quite a chore for a well balanced high self esteem woman who knows what she wants. But what if you were dating a moderate to low self esteemed woman? A woman who had issues and trouble finding herself? You'd probably end up owning a mess, (duh).

This proves the point that a man in search for a mate has to be focused on not only what he wants, but focused on a woman who can handle today's societal stresses of the NWO woman without too much damage.

CHAPTER 6

FINDING THE MATE

Once there was a rich man who had three girlfriends. He wanted to get married but he couldn't decide on which one to marry. To help him in his choice he gave each girlfriend $5,000.00 to whatever they wanted with it.

The first girlfriend spent the money on herself. New clothes, hair, tanning beds etc. When he checked on her she said "I spent the money on making myself more beautiful for you because I love you so much". The rich man was impressed.

The second girlfriend spent her money on gifts for the rich man. She bought him an expensive watch and clothes, etc. When he checked on her she said," I spent the money on you because I love you so much". The rich man was impressed.

The third girlfriend gave the rich man back all of the money he gave her plus a bank book with a $125,000.00 in it. "I invested all the money on stock options and put it in an account with both our names in it because I love you so much". The rich man was impressed.

So which girlfriend did he marry? He married the one with the biggest tits because guys are like that you know.

In business, the military and even in the church, managers will go to extraordinary lengths to find and select the best-qualified person for a particular position. Now take that same person and task him to find a mate for life. What we might see is that he utilized only a small fraction of the criteria and resources at his disposal to find a wife than he did for much less important positions.

BEHIND EVERY GREAT MAN...

When you think about it what is the position of a women relative to a man? Even in the New World Order she's a companion; she's a partner representing the man in the world. A man is judged by the company he keeps, (that especially includes his wife). Have you ever heard the phrase "Isn't that Jim Johnson's wife" with her lovely children? As opposed to "Isn't that Jim Johnson's wife sucking that man's tongue down her throat in the car"? She's the keeper of the nest, (you can have a clean tastefully decorated home or a pig sty with bugs). She can augment your life and career potentiating your efforts or become such a loadstone that you're almost certain to fail in your endeavors. In the business world no boss wants staffers with "problems". If a man is constantly worried about what his wife is doing then he isn't focusing on his job like he should be.

Most importantly she's the other half of your children's genetic makeup and their central development figure. If you choose poorly you can end up with a myriad of problems that will not only plague you in your lifetime but also plague your children and maybe even your grandchildren. You're not only making a decision of love, but a lifetime and "generational' decision that will effect an entire "branch" of your family tree. Considering what's at stake here you might want to rethink and improve your selection process.

IF YOU DON'T KNOW WHAT YOU WANT, (You'll Probably Get Something Else)

The first step in the female selection process is to decide what type of woman you want. Review your personal mission statement. What type of female will assist you in obtaining your desired end-state?

1) Professional
2) Domestic Engineer, (read housewife)
3) General labor, (blue collar worker)
4) Or a hybrid of the first three

The nature of the women that you may have discovered as "the one for you" is critical above all else. This nature is maintained in two categories:

1) What is common to all women.
2) What is specific to the one woman you have focused on.

If you want to be successful you should always refer to your mission statement in your mind throughout the selection process. Always mentally fill out your profile before deciding to commit to a female. Any "warning flags" should be resolved by the time commitment takes place.

THE PARABLE OF THE PORCHE AND THE MINI-VAN

Selecting women is commensurate to selecting cars. Everybody wants a high-speed low drag Porsche that's fast, soooooo sexy and really hot to drive. With that you'd be the envy of all your friends. The down side is that the car is very expensive, insurance is high and the maintenance is crippling at times, (not to mention those tickets). Accessories are a must! If you don't keep these babies tuned just right then they have very poor performance, (if they run at all). Now a Dodge Minivan is a good dependable vehicle, reasonable price, insurance and maintenance. This car kind of sucks to be in unless you're hauling a large amount of people. What you probably need is something in between. Having a super sexy, gorgeous, hot in the sack, babe unit is really really fun. You'd be the envy of all your friends. However, is she the mother of your children? Will she nurture them? Care for you when you're sick? Or will she get bored with you and fuck other men while you're at work? Which one do you want to grow old with? Are you beginning to get the picture?

IF YOU SLEEP WITH DOGS… (You'll Might Get Fleas)

My Father had a rule he told us when we were kids. "Never date a woman you'd be afraid of marrying because you never know when cupid's arrow will strike". Aside from the cupid shit he's right on the money.

This concept is simple; you date a whore, (ho) for fun. You're having a good time screwing her etc. Then find out one fine day that you have fallen in love with her, (or she tells you she's pregnant). Now you're really fucked. If she doesn't magically change her whoring ways to be your Mrs. Whatever you're fucked! Or worse she tries the Mrs. Whatever thing for a while and decides it's not for her. However she likes the kids and the money you bring in. So she just might cheat on you until you catch her. Or she'll just divorce your ass and you can watch your children develop into well-rounded, stable individuals when they see Mommy with the new "friend of the week" or have several different "Step-fathers". The end-state is that you (and you're your children) are fucked. Your options at that point are very limited (unless she really fucks up by the numbers). Simple rule never date a whore! It's that simple. If you just have to… use her for one-night stands, but never more than once or twice, (always use a rubber). Note: Women can still get pregnant when you use a rubber and it's not 100% protection from AIDS either.

THE QUESTIONNAIRE, A BEGINNING OF A PROCESS…

A good technique to find the type of woman you want is the questionnaire. We recommend this type of selection process. Using the questionnaire won't make you out to be a geek. It's not anything you would openly physically use, (using it in public would make you out to be a geek). It's an "in-house" device that helps you judge women in ALL aspects. We can't tell you what the best female is. It depends on your goals, your likes and dislikes. When using the questionnaire realize that you won't get exactly 100% what you list either. This serves as a tool to know what YOU want in a woman. If you don't know what you want you'll probably get something else.

Set out what your perfect mate should be like. Be very specific! This is a potential partner for the rest of your life, the mother of your children and the owner of half of your fortune. The questionnaire should be divided into several major subjects. You can change the questioner to suit your preferences. A sample is:

1. Current status.
2. Children.
3. Physical attributes.
4. Nationality
5. Ethics/beliefs.
6. Personality
7. Vices.
8. Entertainment
9. Physical fitness

1. The first issue is the female's status.
    a. Married. Stop right there. No need to go any further. They fuck up your Chi, they have lots of baggage, lots of drama and sometimes they can get you shot, (not a joke). Major point Is She has no honor or sense of commitment. How could you ever trust her? Hunting a married woman is not honorable. Never be the "transitional man". It almost always ends up in disaster.

       War Story. A co-worker worked with this married woman for two years. He realized that although attracted to this woman he was forced to respect the matrimonial boundaries. For 2 ½ years they worked together while she whined daily about her "fuck stick" husband. This guy had a poor work history, chain smoker and spent his free time on the internet "dark side" of porn. A platonic relationship developed and eventually she announces to him that she's wants to leave her husband. This starts a new type of relationship that began on a physical dimension and ended up in a love relationship. The sex was dripping hot and he was patiently waiting for her to "get free" seeing her in stolen moments. Weeks turned into to months and after six months of an emotional roller coaster she tells him that she can't leave her husband. It would be too hard on the kids and she really wants her marriage to work out blah, blah, blah, bullshit, bullshit, bullshit... So they split and the guy ended up getting trashed. She got a great "Fantasy Island" episode from the whole thing. Now they have to continue to work together making life hard for all who have to work next to them. The "Transitional Man". When women are cheating, recently separated or newly divorced they tend to date a "transitional man". This is usually a quick choice, a fantasy or someone in close proximity and/or anonymity. They could also sub-consciously use you as a vehicle to "escape" her current relationship. Rarely do they ever culminate in a true committed relationship. If they do have a relationship it usually falls short of everybody's expectations and ends up in disaster. If you're "really most sincerely" attracted to a woman then wait and try to date her after a while.

b. Engaged. Same as above.
c. Separated. Don't actively date, but get her number. She's on the hunt. She's not single but testing the waters of the single life. If you're out for a piece of ass fine. If you're looking for a partner leave it lie, if you do pick her up feed her with a very long spoon. Many women "reconcile" after a while. Typically this is an emotionally charged period for both partners of the marriage. The man sees his wife out with another man and "flips out" occasionally ending in violence, (It has happened many times). Whether or not they're newly divorced or separated, it is very wise to stay away from this situation. Warning: The potential for "vortex behavior" is very high here, (see next section).

The Grudge Fuck. This is an important concept for you can stumble on to it easily and end up in shit soup if not prepared. Sometimes women when hurt, by an unscrupulous fuck-stick or dumped, will want to get even by fucking somebody. This can be a woman who has no intention of leaving her husband/boyfriend. Or she has left him and wants "pay back" for the pain she experienced from his indiscretions/actions. It can remain an anonymous experience or she can fuck you and tell her partner. The scenarios are dangerous and many. Some women will even have sex with the fuck-sticks best friend or even a brother to get even. This is obviously a really sick bitch and it's best to keep your distance.

d. Divorced. "How long" is the main question here. Newly divorced females, (NDF) are either needy as hell or bitches. They can be a great source of wild sex if you're just on the hunt. The NDF seems to have an un-satiable appetite to re-validate her sexual desirability. Never actively date until divorced for at least two years.
e. Widowed. This is sad but men die and they leave widows. This can be good or it can be bad depending on the particular circumstances. If he was a fantastic husband, provider and she dated him since high school it could be rough. You could always be compared to him forever, (it would be like living with him but he never does anything wrong). Keep in mind the time since his demise; are you the first man she's dated? Has she "let go" of her dead husband?
f. Single. Best option overall. How long has she been single, (If you're looking at a woman in her late 30's early 40's and she's never been married look hard at her personality)? When was her last relationship? Has she just broken up with her lover? Why did they break up? Did she live with a guy? Was she "pseudo married"? Why did she never get married? Was she a "party girl"?

Now you're not going to ask all of these questions prior to the first date. Not even in the first date. But you should try to obtain this information in the first three dates, (along with all the other information). If you've dated through friends then you can get a wealth of information from the friends prior to the date. This section is rather important.

THE VORTEX SYNDROME

During the initial dating period some women will attempt to cloud negative issues or hide deficiencies by using outstanding sex or victim status. This used to be called "pussy brain". Basically the woman fucks you out of your sanity. While you're spinning around in a sexual haze you don't pay close attention to the facts. Don't get sucked into what we call the "vortex of the victim" and/or the "vortex of outstanding sex".

Men get bombarded with the "saving syndrome" in the media and women exploit it whenever it's beneficial for them, (which is 90% of the fucking time).

Example: Watch Richard Gere and Julia Roberts in the movie "Pretty Woman". Roberts is a prostitute,(victim of an unscrupulous society), Gere, (a millionaire who is a product of the same unscrupulous society) "saves" her taking her off the street eventually wanting her to be his mistress. She declines stating that she wants the "fairytale" where the Knight rides up in his horse, climbs the tower and saves her ass. He does "save" her and they both live happily ever after.

In reality Gere would have to be a real psycho to want some $100 whore off the street steaming with disease, drugs and God knows whatever when he could afford to buy a high class $10,000 a night educated "companion" who would jump at the chance to be his mistress. But the main point here is that women are indoctrinated by the media to be "victims" and men are equally brainwashed to be their "rescuers", (see the nature of men).

2) Vortex of the Victim. The use of the victim strategy is well used and very successful. By claming victim status the female can easily explain all sorts of poor behavior away.
   Example. "Well, I started drinking/doing coke because of the physical abuse/drugs I had to endure with my last boyfriend/husband". Or "My husband was so mentally abusive to me I became depressed and that's why I'm taking Prozac and Xanax". If she has her act rehearsed well and applies some good sex the guy will probably believe it. Most men will immediately want to "rush to the rescue. Why? Because it's in our nature, Luke Skywalker HAS to save Princess Leia.
3) Vortex of Outstanding Sex. This is where the woman sexually takes you to places you only dreamed about. Some people call it "movie sex" because it answers so many of your fantasies. It starts off very hot and steamy. Your mesmerized, transfixed by the shear pleasure and quantity of talk about sex, (talk about sex is the sex you and your buddies bragged or fantasized about).

Sometimes women will use the "vortex" to hold on to a man. She might do this if she's insecure in her own self-worth/self-esteem. She might not feel she is "good enough" for her man and will compensate by giving him fantasy sex, (threesomes, group or swinging). This must be looked at as a potential major self-esteem co-dependency issue. Look very closely if you see this and date for a long time.

Actions on the objective. Always delay sex for a while to dispassionately feel her out, (mentally not physically). This tack will make her think your special, (especially when you're not trying to race into a relationship and the sack). It'll also make her put forth more effort if she thinks she hasn't branded you with her camel toe. Keep your head, (the big one) in the game and dispassionately start to sort this out. She's going to try and lead you from the facts with the vortexes. She can use them singularly or in concert. She's either covering something up or trying to get you addicted to her pussy, (See the "camel toe chronicles"). Try to be aloof and act like you have a purpose. You like her but you're still a mystery. Even if you're smitten please don't show it now dummy. All pussy will get old regardless of whom you're fucking and how great it is. The key is to find a woman you can have a good relationship with. Once the sex is over you still have to talk to her. You might find that life with Bambi isn't so fantastic.

2. Children. Another VERY IMPORTANT section. This should be determined early in the dating process, (like in the first 7 dates). If there's a wide chiasm between your plans and hers then get the hell out now. MAJOR ISSUE.
    a. Dose she like children? Some women will have children, but not really like them. This would leave a lot of the parenting to you. It might also fuck up your children. Expose her to some children a few times. Watch her reaction and the children's reaction. Children are usually hard to fool when it comes to imposters. Possible deal breaker.
    b. Does she have children? Remember the older you get before you settle down increases the probability of hooking up with a female who already has children. Does this suit your plans and your time line? War-game her children into your mission statement/plan. How does it affect your goals? Also look at her parenting techniques. Do they match with what you expect in a mother.

Note: When determining the age to have your children. Always add 20 years to your present age.

Example: I'm only 35 so I have plenty of time to have kids. Wrong again. When you look at the total picture you're 55 years old. That's the age you'll be before you're through raising children and will be functionally free to travel, retire etc. That can also be the age you're through paying child support. You don't want to be 69 years old and still having to shit out child support on a fixed income. You'll suffer and so will your kids, (unless of course you're filthy rich).

War Story. I dated this woman who had a 2 ½ year old child. We got along swimmingly but she had this policy about disciplining her child, (actually there was no fucking policy at all). I was of the belief that children should be well behaved. This kid was totally out of control and I eventually said something to her. She was irate at having me comment on her child. We finally ended the relationship because of the child.

Is the child psycho? Yes sometimes children can be psycho. This can be familial, (inherited) or it just happens, (mutation of some gene in the fetal development process etc.). Whatever the reason is the kids fucked up mentally. You need to get a full understanding of what the kid's problems are before you decide to commit. If possible try and ascertain what the Mother's mental status is before you decide to make anymore children. Remember children with problems = you with problems.

War Story. One of my best friends married a woman with a troubled child. Initially the problems were small, (acting out in grade school, belligerent attitude, etc.). As the child grew so did his problems. Now the child is in his early teens and is still acting out but in a big way. Recently he had attacked his Mother and Grandmother with rocks, broke up the house ending in a clash with the police. Now he's in all sorts of expensive anger management counseling, psychiatric counseling and possibly an institution, (read really fucking expensive) and if that doesn't work juvenal detention camp with foster home placement. My best friend is pulling his hair out worrying about his other children in the house with

this mini-Hannibal Lecther throwing fits all over the place and trying to pay for all of this shit. His relationship with his wife is also strained because her "chi" is all fucked up over the potential outcome of her first born.
Situations like this can mushroom into much larger ones. It can also break up a marriage leaving YOUR children in the hands of... whatever. This is an important MAJOR issue. Your eyes need to be completely open to evaluate this objectively. Don't let the Mom give you the situation, (she'll gloss it over out of loyalty to her child). Do your own homework and objectively appraise the situation before making a decision. Strong potential for Vortex behavior.

c. If she has children, what is her "ex-" like? Something that is frequently NOT looked at is the "ex-". Is he cool? Is he actively involved in the children (s) lives? Does he pay child support? Is he psycho? All of these are really semi-major to major issues. For example:
    i. Is he cool with the fact that you're in the picture "fucking his wife" in front of his kids? Some guys have a tough time letting go. They can stalk you, start fights, show up at the bar where you hang out. Sometimes it can be a lot of "drama". They can also inflict all sorts of shit on you through the children. Statements like "My dad says I don't have to do what you tell me to do" or "Daddy says you took mommy away from him so we can't be a family anymore", (welcome to fuck stick world in the eyes of a six year old). The possibilities for disaster are as endless as the stars in the skies.
    ii. Is the father "active" in his children's lives. Does he show up for events? If he doesn't are the kids' Chi all fucked up about it? Many problems with kids arise from the father not giving a shit.
    iii. Child support. This may sound hard, but the facts are clear. Does he pay his share? If you're divorced and have to pay your share so should he. Especially if you're looking at multiple children. Clothing, food, medical care, fun and college will drain away your early retirement dreams. The fuck stick on the other hand is having a good time

since he doesn't have to pay shit. Also you have to ask yourself "Does she want me for support or for real love"? Major issue.

iv. Being psycho. They're out there. The ones who are more than a ½ a bubble off plum. They're the ones that purposely fuck the kids up to get to the ex-wife. They're the ones that drive around drunk with the two year old driving your wife insane with worry.

War Story. Ben married this wonderful woman with a little girl. She was divorced from this psycho alcoholic for 3 years when they met. After her marriage to Ben the ex- decides to re-claim his daughter. This man is a bonified psycho/ alcoholic. Two counts of DUI and an assault with jail time at the county. After a court battle, (read lots of cash spent) the court ruled to allow the father reasonable visitation. Since he had paid his time for the assault and DUI they could see no reason not to let him have her. My buddies wife played by the rules, let the fuck stick have her and then listened to her recount the stories of how she spent her Saturday in the bar with her dad while he watched sports and drank. They tried to stop him two more times, (read lots more cash) and only eventually stopped him after he got a DUI with her in the car. Then he could still see her except that he couldn't drive her,(now his girl friend picks her up). Throughout the marriage they have fought with this psycho and they have lost.

When the female presents with children then you have to consider the total "entertainment" package. It's not a showstopper, but you must look at it all. Don't get caught into the "vortex of the victim". This is easy to do when they appear to be so weak and helpless, (while fucking you like a porn star).

d. Does she want children? If your plan calls for some, and she doesn't want any dump her now. There are too many women out there who want kids.

e. Does she "Can't wait to have children?" If she's a beaming bouncing young woman with the baby bug WATCH OUT!

These women have a high probability of "birth control accidents".

   a. If yes to children, how many does she want? Another high priority area. You might want two; she might be a strict Catholic who only believes in the "rhythm method" (also known as "Vatican roulette") for birth control who really wants six or seven kids. Find out early. Don't easily accept her agreements. High probability for really most sincerely "birth control accidents".
   b. Birth control. How does she feel about "vasectomy vs. tubal legation"? You can slip this into many conversations if you're good. Watch her reaction.

f. Physical attributes. This is pretty easy because you can see most of it. We're picking our perfect woman. We can list anything we want:
   a. Height.
   b. Hair color.
   c. Eye color.
   d. Build.
      i. Petite
      ii. Slender
      iii. Well built
      iv. Muscular/Athletic
      v. Full figured, (FAT)
      vi. Jabba the Gut, (really most sincerely fat)

g. Ethnic background.
   a. Nationality. You wouldn't think this would be a serious issue, but meet an Islamic woman in the U.S. or a Jewish woman when you're a gentile. Some families practically disown a child if they marry outside their religion. SEMI-MAJOR ISSUE.
   b. Ethnic features. This is a physical preference only. Minor issue.
   c. Cultural responsibilities. In some cultures the children are brought up to keep the parents and support them. Not a showstopper, but you want to know this going onto the relationship not when

you get engaged or are married. Semi-major issue.

h. Ethics/beliefs.
    a. Religion. More relationships have been trashed secondary to the "R" issue than any other. They say never to discuss religion but you have to do it sometime. The sooner you find this out the better. This is a 3d or 4th date issue; find out if your religion and her religion are compatible. It would be better to dump her early than when you're in love with her. MAJOR ISSUE.
    b. Religious responsibilities. Like the cultural responsibilities above, some religions have certain responsibilities like making sure the children are raised in that religion. You need to know this relatively early to make your decision. SEMI-MAJOR issue.

War Story. I dated this Indian girl named Rapauli. She was gorgeous and we were fantastic together. Everything was perfect until we started talking about children and religion. I was in favor of letting the kids see both religions and choosing when they became of age. She was adamant that they be raised Hindu, (that's what she was). We argued this for almost a year and only had to break up in the end. Both of us had broken hearts but it was our only choice.

    c. Children's religion. As above, what religion are you? If that differs from your wife's then what religion is your children? Important matters to know about before the commitment. SEMI-MAJOR ISSUE.
    d. Enthusiasm. Healthy amount of enthusiasm can indicate a good self esteem, and productive. Too much can make you wonder if she has personality disorders, (like bi-polar and Manic Depressive). Refer to Chapter 3 Self esteem. Minor issue.
    e. Negativity. How does she see the world? Is the glass always ½ full? If this is the case you'll be always fighting an uphill battle. Semi-Major issue.

f. Political persuasion. The potential exists that many fights can take place over conservative vs. liberal views. It can range from the political arena to child rearing and general life issues. SEMI-MAJOR Issue.

g. Spiritual. Nice to know but check for being "too far out on a limb". Always remember she is your ambassador to the world, (both social and business). Minor issue.

War story. Paul had met Barbara at a restaurant. She was a massage therapist and he was a physical therapist. It was lust at first sight. Everything was perfect. Barb lived in a neighboring city. After a few dates Paul went to see her when she dropped the "disclosure" on him. She told him that she was a WICCA practitioner. This is about a ½ step from witchcraft in many peoples eyes. Paul decided that this WICCA was too OTBT, (off the beaten trail) religion wise to handle. Again moderation of everything is the key, including religion.

h. Superstitious. A little bit is fun, a lot starts to suck. If she's too far out there then dump her. This can easily lead to the "dark side" of religion. Major Issue.

i. Personality.
    a. Feminine or macho. If she's very "macho" acting you could have trouble establishing the "Alpha Dog" leadership position. It could also indicate "other" lifestyle desires, (closet lesbian?). The again she could just be a "bitch". Minor issue.
    b. Caring. This is an important item. It's a natural component for women. When it's missing it could indicate developmental or self-esteem problems. Semi-major issue.
    c. Supportive. Does she have the necessary temperament to be a supportive partner? You'll have many goals in your life and to have a non-supporting person along would be like dragging a lot of "dead weight" around. Minor issue.

d. Aggressive/competitive. Someaggressiveness is good, too much is bad. It can hinder Alpha dog goals and cause "competition" between you and your spouse. Competition is good in the work force but bad at the home front. Semi-major issue.
e. Warm. Friendly, Congenial with nice smile is always beneficial. Remember she will be your ambassador in the community. Minor issue.
f. Understanding. This is a temperament issue. Minor issue.
g. Loving. We've noticed that some women aren't loving individuals. Despite good looks, despite good job a woman without the capacity to SHOW, (she may actually love you) love could eventually alienate you and ruin the marriage, (dependent on your needs). SEMI-MAJOR issue.
h. Patient. Important issue. This is necessary for good child development. It's also necessary for us men who from time to time fuck up. SEMI-MAJOR issue.
i. Flexible. How does she cope with changes in plans? Fucked up plans is unavoidable in life. Does she fall apart if a plan doesn't come off like she wants it? Or does she "adjust fire and continue on? How a person reacts to these "little upsets" is important. Minor issue.
j. % of energy. No Sloths please. This can be serious for couples. Another "dead weight issue". If you notice her with poor energy look for long term trends of low energy. If no long term low energy then think possible depression. Typically you don't get more energy as you get older, (you get less). SEMI-MAJOR issue.
k. Drive and ambition. This is good within reason. Too much can lead to mixed up family mission statement/goals. Also competition can develop. Semi-major issue.

l. Bearing. How does she present herself? Does she appear confident, calm and collected? Or does look timid, shy and withdrawn? Does she meet your eyes when you talk to her? Remember the old saying: "How she walks determines her work". Minor issue.
m. Angry. If she has a bad temper with a hair trigger then DUMP HER!!! You have no time to spend on this type of woman. Severe anger at others will eventually be turned on you. MAJOR issue!

War Story. I had dated this girl in Augusta, GA. She was a striking blonde, thin very fit and well educated. While seriously dating her I noticed was that she had this seething temper she would let loose at her ex-husband, (it was almost like a fit). Once her temper was started she fed it with gasoline until it literally "burned itself out". Our relationship was racing along, sex was fantastic and we were getting very close to the commitment stage. One night we had a minor confrontation and she let her temper loose at me. We were in bed after sex when it happened. I thought for a long while and then got up and went home. As I left she asked, "If I shut the fuck up will you stay?" I never called her again. Why? Because I didn't want to deal with the excessive temper she could deal out. The relationship was relatively new and the cost of the loss was negligible.

Remember: The temper she gives others will = the temper she gives you eventually!

n. Jealously. Jealously is the primary symptom of abusive relationships. It's also a core component of sexual addictions and love addiction. Everybody get a little jealous. Again look for the moderate vs: the pathological. Moderate is okay, pathological is really fucking bad. MAJOR issue. Dump the bitch!

War Story. Greg and Deborah dated for two years. During this time she had been insanely jealous and possessive. This jealously eventually developed into a couple of physically abusive episodes. Greg finally got tired of the "shit train" and broke it off. One night Deborah broke the window of his house and climbed in to catch Greg with a wet dick slicing her leg up in the process. Obviously Greg had to call the Police who arrested Deborah after she went to the hospital to sew up her leg. The girl Greg was fucking, (and really liked) was traumatized to the extent that she didn't want to see him anymore (since she feared for her life from his crazy ex-girlfriend). After that Greg had his car "keyed" three times and had hundreds of crank phone calls. She would show up at the same bars causing scenes and fights. She was operating an emotional terrorism program against him. In retrospect he thought the jealously was cool initially, (wow she really fucking digs me). But it grew in intensity and severity culminating in to a violent scenario. He eventually had to leave the area since this bitch wouldn't leave his ass alone.

o. Confident. Some is good, too much is dangerous. Look for the signs. Too little look for self-esteem issues. Minor issue.
p. Successful. Always a good thing, watch for over confidence. Successful women tend to be bitches. They seem to have trouble switching to their "feminine" side because their male side works so well for them. This could be serious trouble for a man who's intent on establishing the "alpha Dog" in a relationship. It takes a special woman to handle success and be a good wife. MAJOR ISSUE.
q. Introverted or extroverted. These are potential pathological manifestations of poor self-esteem. Introverted possible self esteem issues, extroverted possible bi-polar. Issues. You should examine very hard prior to commitment. Look for the "pathological" levels of each type. Semi-major issue.
r. Sincere. Do we need a woman who isn't sincere? Will she be prone to telling lies to you and your children? This is self-explanatory. Fake women, fake stories… faked orgasms. Semi-major issue.
s. Passionate. This is a personal preference issue. Some men like it hot. Some men couldn't care

less. We have found that the really fucking hot ones also have more maintenance issues. The other issue is sex eventually gets old with the same woman. If she's a hottie in bed it certainly does help. Always remember that it took a lot of "practice" for her to get to that level of "expertise". It's been our experience that the hotter a woman is the crazier she is. Look for a middle of the road chick. Some passion some calmness. Semi-major issue.

t. Independent. This is a double-edged sword. Men like independent women. However too independent leads to poor bonding of the man and woman. Also you have to ask why is she so independent? Does she have "trust issues" secondary to self esteem concerns? Again some independence is good too much will cause you to look deeper. Semi-major issue.

u. Sense of humor. This is always fun. It makes for a fun time. Too serious of a woman leads to boredom with her. Again a little humor is good, too much and you might think she's craving the attention. Will she make a good wife if she craves the attention of a crowd? Think your goals and what you want out of a mate.

v. FAITHFUL. DUH! If she's not 100% of this DUMP HER IMMEDIATELY. This is an Ethics/Values/Integrity,(EVI) issue. Don't hesitate to think about it and definitely don't date her to fuck. You have selected her for qualities of a potential mate. You could easily fall in love with her. We can't think of a more important issue. Warning Will Robinson Whore alert, whore alert!!!!!!!!!!!! MAJOR MAJOR MAJOR ISSUE!!!!!

w. Romantic. As with the passion this is personally up to you. Right now you want to fuck. As you get older you'll want some romance to add ambience to your fucking. Minor issue.

x. Pride in appearance. Remember she's your ambassador to the community. If she looks like shit then you look like shit. It can also be an indicator of poor self-esteem. If she takes no pride in her appearance then do you think she'll take any pride in how her house looks? How your children look? Is she a "neat freak? That could be a pain in the ass. Look at her house/apartment. Is it messy? Is it dirty? Look in places where she wouldn't normally clean. Major issue.

y. General intellect. Bambi or Madam Currie you take your choice. The sex will get old we promise you. Whatever will you do with a stupid shallow woman then? You're going to have to talk to her. You could have a boring life, (unless you like to watch cartoons and sitcoms). You could get rid of her but why go through all that? Tits will sag, the face will wrinkle and the pussy juice will dry up eventually. But the mind is the last to go. Major issue.

z. Compassionate. We think this is important. Compassion is one of the windows to the entire personality. If she has poor to little compassion we feel that she wouldn't be able to love very well either. Major issue.

aa. Gentile. Some men like them prissy, some like them rough. This is a personal choice. Minor issue.

bb. Cautious. Some caution is good, too much indicates possible self esteem issues. Look for excessive amounts. Minor issue.

cc. Deep. Again Bambi or Condelezza Rice. Your choice. But for reasons listed above we recommend you to consider the mind as well as the physical. Semi-major issue.

dd. Careful. Look to cautious above. Minor issue.

ee. Sexy. MAJOR ISSUE. This can easily make or break a relationship. Even though it's wrong spiritually, check her out. Look for normal drives and technique. Watch out for the vortex of great sex. Great sex can equal lots of practice with many men. If she's dead in the water and you don't like humping a piece of dead meat, then dump her immediately. This is cruel but necessary. MAJOR ISSUE.

War Story. John is a dentist. He hired this blond for his office. Eventually the human element took over and a relationship was started. What was so fantastic was that this woman had John so wrapped around her finger she had never had sex with him until their wedding night, (they dated for two years). Now this wasn't a blushing bride either. She was divorced for 3 years. Now once married she gave him sporadic sex, (usually given up with a fight) and he reported it sucked badly. She had immediately gotten pregnant during the honeymoon. Now he's stuck for a while in a real shitty relationship. TRY BEFORE YOU BUY.

ff. Sexually adventurous. Is she willing to "spice up" the sex to keep it interesting when it starts to get old? Some is good, too much isn't. Watch for women who like it "too spiced up", this can lead to the dark side of sex. If she wants to swing from the chandelier during sex rethink your choice. Semi-major issue.

gg. Reliable. You want a woman who "says what she means and means what she says". Dependability and reliability are the traits you're looking for in a wife and a mother. This fosters trust. Semi-major issue.

hh. Selfish. Major issue for us. Selfish women fly so many warning flags! A selfish woman will plague you forever. They can even get selfish with their children. Not something you want. Dump immediately. MAJOR ISSUE!!!!!

ii. Proud. Proud is good so long as it's within reason. A person has to be able to admit to being wrong every now and then. Many disasters started because people were too proud to admit they're wrong. Semi-major issue.

jj. Willpower. This is good. Will power to get her through a lonely week while you're on a business trip or on a military deployment. IT does carry a double edge sword if she ever decides to hold out for sex. Minor issue.

kk. On time. Minor issue. It's nice to have but not a major showstopper. Observe for major events she really wants though. If she's late for those then she might have severe time management problems. Try to fix before you buy. Minor issue.

j. Vices.
    a. Smoking
        i. She loves it, sucks to be you
        ii. She enjoys it, sucks to be you
        iii. She smokes socially, (like with drinking), barely tolerable
        iv. She never smokes, our personal choice. Remember that a smoker is a smoker is a smoker. Meaning that very few women can quit smoking for good. Most will give it up for your love. But as soon as they feel comfortable with your love they'll pick it back up again, (usually after some stressful event). If your mate smokes then you have to deal with it. Love her with smoking or leave her. Whatever is your decision you have to live with it. If you take her smoking then you have to live with it. There's no bitching after the fact. This is your time to choose now. MAJOR ISSUE.
    b. Drinking.
        i. Love it? Danger Will Robinson... Warning... Warning, Dump this bitch and quick, (Unless you like doing the 12 steps of AA). People who love to drink and do so frequently will usually get worse. They're probably already addicted to it. Dump the bitch. MAJOR ISSUE.
        ii. Enjoy it. What kind of a woman really enjoys drinking? It isn't a fucking sport or an advocation! If she 'enjoys it" too much then treat as above. Don't waste time on this relationship. Dump the bitch. MAJOR ISSUE.

iii. Social drinker. Acceptable. Monitor her when she's out with her friends. If she hangs out with friends who really drink a lot then she might be drinking a lot too. She might be "putting her best foot forward" and holding back for your benefit. MAJOR ISSUE.

iv. Tea totaler. Why? Never had or had too much at one time? Was she the main entertainment event at a frat party when she drank too much? She could have had a Daddy who drinks too much. Could be an indicator of poor self-esteem. Find out! Semi-Major issue.

v. Post rehab. Do we really have to explain this? Date at your own considerable risk dummy. MAJOR MAJOR ISSUE!!!!!!!

c. Drugs

Ever tried? What type? How much? How long? How long ago? Anything more than pot DUMP THE BITCH. Drugs have a way getting into a person and destroying everything it touches. Speed can permanently damage your heart. Cocaine dominates your life, (crack included). LSD can permanently change your DNA structure. You don't have time to waste on women like this. Dating a woman like this is an extreme long shot. . Some physicians claim that only 5% of truly committed drug addicts ever get the Monkey of their back.

<<<<Warning>>>> Beware of the 'Vortex of the Victim". Do not get drawn into this! People who are actively into drugs have a steamer trunk full of monumental issues. This would swallow up your time and resources. You'd never have a guarantee of freedom from it. MAJOR MAJOR ISSUE.

War Story. Courtney was an RN at a hospital. She was beautiful, competent and very sexy. She was everything a guy would want. Except that she had a slight issue. She was addicted to drugs. So much that she was stealing them from the hospital where she worked. She was dating another RN, (Mark) who tried in vein to get her to quit. She'd been to rehab twice and failed. Mark followed her around hospital to hospital trying to get her to quit. He finally found her high as shit fucking some derelict. He finally dumped her but wasted three years of his life and a shit-load of cash trying to get her to stay sober. She finally lost her license to practice.

i. Light drugs. Pot can be okay depending on your preferences. We don't advocate it. Pot is great for someone you're gonna PARTY with dude and later fuck. But for the mother of your children??? DUMP THE BITCH. MAJOR ISSUE.

ii. Post rehab. No brainer here. Roughly 5% of the really most sincerely rehab drug users ever break the habit of serious drugs, (coke, heroin and crack). It's a gamble at best so why date someone like this unless you're really hard up or stupid, (we're sorry we're so insensitive … not!). They're too many non-drug women out there. Sorry ex-druggers, but we're giving our readers the best advice we can. Sucks to be you! DUMP THE BITCH. MAJOR MAJOR ISSUE.

iii. Never. Best choice. Our personal recommendation.

d. Sexual aberrations.

i. Free sexual entity/awareness. Reads whore. DUMP THE BITCH. MAJOR ISSUE.

ii. Swings. Reads whore with a pervert for a partner. MAJOR ISSUE. If you like this shit then you need counseling sicko! DUMP THE BITCH.

iii. Closet lesbian, (or previous lesbian relationship). Possible psych issues. True lesbians don't have anything to hide. They're proud of their choice and usually don't give a shit who knows. High possibility of self-esteem damage. She obviously doesn't know what she wants. Also possibility of her "rediscovering" herself later and taking your children to live with her lover "Miss Crunchbull". What a way to develop your son. Sucks to be you. DUMP THE BITCH. MAJOR ISSUE.

iv. Lesbian. Cool … party on Garth! (Just joking) Again if she's a true lesbian then she shouldn't be with you. True love doesn't conquer all. She's obviously really fucking confused about her sexual choices. You don't need confused women. Why do you need to waste your time? Dump the bitch after you have a three some with her, (just joking).

v. Normal sexual practices. Our choice for long-term stability.

This is complete a list as we can develop. You can add more or take away at your discretion. The key issue is the mental checklist you have developed in your head about what you want. We have also given you guidance about what you don't want in a generic sense.

Let's Play….RATE THE TRAIT

Once you have made a list of all the desirable traits are regarding the "perfect" mate, you go get her right? No, to think that you'd find a woman will ALL of your wants is unrealistic. What you must do now is prioritize these traits for YOU. What are the really important aspects you HAVE to have vs. those aspects you'd WISH she had vs. what aspects you really don't care about. Here's our sample list:

Height	5'9"
Nationality	American
Color	Dark Brown
Eyes	Blue
Weight	120 lbs
Build	36 24 33
Educational level	college grad
Previous marriages	none
Children	none
Religion	Catholic
Salary	$50,000+
Personality	calm
Work ethic	good
Mental history	none
Temper	none

This is a short list but we're just trying to teach you the process. You now assign priorities to each item of your list. Assign one to ten to each of your mating criteria regarding its importance to you, (this is a personal thing). Let's take another look at our list with the priorities added.

Height	5'9"	2
Nationality	American	2
Color	Dark Brown	2
Eyes	Blue	2
Weight	120 lbs	7
Build	36 24 33	5
Educational level	college grad	9
Previous marriages	none	4
Children	none	6
Religion	Catholic	10
Salary	$50,000+	5
Personality	calm	7
Work ethic	good	4
Mental history	none	10
Temper	none	5

We are starting to develop a complete picture of what we want in a woman. Since we've been raised Catholic, then we place a very high priority on the girl being Catholic. We also have a high emphasis on educational level. So we are developing a "profile" for the perfect mate. We know what we definitely don't want is a non-catholic or a mental case. That's the rule, but it's not cut in stone either. Remember this is a guide; you can leave the path for some things.

Once your list is complete, do you run around all the bars with a copy of your profile? No, but this tool will help YOU to know what YOU want! All men young or old should have this written down in their head a profile of what they're looking for. It's like that old saying "If you don't know where you're going…you'll probably end up somewhere else". Have at least an idea what you want in life when it comes to women. Note: Discovery of all traits with a priority greater than "7" should be obtained before the 7th date.

Age. This should be in your profile but we have elected to talk about it separately. Age should never matter. Now that is once again so much shit! Age does matter. Hook up with a woman 10 years older and you get a ragged older woman at 60 while you're able to get a 35 year old when your 50. You'll be hit with daily temptations to cheat or leave her. God forbid you go into court with a female judge when you want to dump your "old squeeze", (emphasis on old). Now the other way is stupid as well. Don't be 40 and date a 20 year old for a relationship. She'll eventually dump your ass, take your kids and fuck a younger man. You don't want to share your fortune with her either. The best age range is five years up ten years down. Go over that and you're in the trouble zone.

WHY DO WOMEN WANT TO COMMIT

Why do women even bother to commit? After reading our book many men might wonder why do we commit? Like the geese that flies south in the winter, most of us will take a woman and make a family. It follows the natural progression of life and is in our male nature. Let's look into why a woman would want to commit to you. Women in general have a myriad of reasons to nest with a particular man. The least of these reasons is sex. Women can get sex anywhere anytime and anyplace. Women will date a man for some of the following reasons:

1. Love/family. This is a good reason for initiating a relationship. The woman has been to college, started her job and is now ready to think about that special guy leading up to the top of the women's love pyramid; marriage. This would eventually lead to children

and so on and so on. This is the fairytale that all of us want to believe.

2. Economic survival. Some women realize that they are not the savvy businesswomen they would have liked to have been. Matter of fact they don't really like the get up in the morning to the alarm clock roaring thing. They would prefer to be the Volvo station wagon types with the 2.5 children and the chocolate lab in the back. These women are out there; the smart ones go to college to find the "right boy". The "duller knives in the drawer work a lack luster job hanging out in bars looking for "Mr. Perfect, but settling for Mr. Kind of, sort of maybe" or "Mr. Close To". Some of these women will do almost anything to obtain financial security. These are the dangerous ones because they are most likely to have birth control "accidents". They have low drive, unhappy with themselves and will blame you for their lot in life. They will be the depressed ones, the ones who will loose the luster of life and drag you off the high road to your success and into the ditches and alleys of fruitless pursuits. Again I'm not saying this is a postulate. Not all less than brilliant women are this way. It just means if you find a woman who happens to fit this profile then you just look a little harder at her and dig a little deeper to check her sincerity and her mental state.
3. The storm damaged boat. If you are an average guy and someday come upon a woman whom you know is way beyond your reach then read the warning flags? I'm not saying don't try to get the best deal you can, but the old saw says," If it's too good to be true, it usually is". When some women get out into the emotional ocean and get ravaged by a few men they are too emotionally drained to compete in the world. They need an "emotional dry-dock" for which they can make "repairs". Now this isn't a conscious thought that they plan, it's just what happens sometimes. They have been in a couple or several failed relationships. They have put all of their emotional coins into fast men or bad boys they thought they could change. They get beat up, financially raped and emotionally exhausted. Consequently they look for a safe harbor to rest and repair. Since all men love to save and fix things they scoop these women up with relish. These women readily accept the tow to calm waters and bask in the emotional safety of their new host. What typically happens is love occurs, marriage and eventually children arrive. The woman then having experienced the joys of all of this becomes recharged and starts to yearn for the open

ocean again. This she does with her children, half of the house, savings and child support. Occasionally they return if they get damaged again but will never be truly happy in your harbor.

"Never Truly Happy Women. A "Never truly happy "woman is someone that no matter what a man does for her in life he will never make her truly happy. She is internally "unhappy". The net result is like swimming with a heavy weight on your back. You expend an enormous amount of energy and don't get very far. These women in their pursuit of "their" happiness lead you all over the map of life. If you try to get them on a common course for the sake of the family boat, they look at you as the reason or focal point of their failure to get to Xanadu. Even when they dump your ass and are free, they'll still blame you because YOU you dumb son-of–a–bitch tricked them into marring you and ruining their life. Either way you're fucked! Your only real counter for this type of woman is recognition of the sub-species and run like hell. This is hard to do when you have a Cindy Crawford look-a –like who fucks you like a nymph. Look for possible borderline personality and strong use of Vortex behavior".

WARNING SIGNS

Let's say you have met a girl that meets approximately 70% of your prioritized "dream girl" criteria. She's good looking and the sex is really fantastic. Are you in the relationship Nirvana yet? Not quite yet grasshopper. While dating her, look for the "warning signs". Warning signs are just what they say. Actions that set off a warning in your brain or our book. Some of these are:

1. Divorced. This is a static warning sign, (if you didn't know earlier). You will probably find this little fact out during the first three dates. Women typically don't let this out immediately. There use to be a severe stigma on divorced people. It's still there, but to a much lesser degree. For you it's not a deal breaker, but should send you to explore more than the never been married girl. Once out in the open she will probably tell you the story, unless it's too "painful", (watch the "too painfuls" it could be a subterfuge for a real screw-up). She will probably tell you "he" was some sort of a fuck stick; abuser, or a homo… whatever. You have to determine the validity of her statement. Always keep in the back of your mind what would make a woman leave the holy grail of relationship states. She was there; she had her "Mrs." Whatever

status and now she's left it probably saying she was a VICTIM. Poor poor pitiful me, feel sorry for me, protect me, love me, take care of me, me, me, me, me... This is why we tell you to look real hard before you leap and date for a long time.

2. The No-fault Divorced Woman. Now when a woman tells you "we just decided to split", is a very serious warning sign. Women who have no reason for divorce (other than to say they were bored with marriage or their spouse) have only one option: run away!!! These are typically people who have no core values regarding the institution of marriage. Commitment to someone or something doesn't exist for them. They're members of "Captain Id's Pleasure Rangers" and live for the moment. Their pleasure is everything. Unfortunately when they marry and have children they try to commit but soon become, bored, unhappy and must move on,(did we mention taking your children and child support with them).
   Note: Captain Id's Pleasure Rangers refers loosely to Freudian psychology dealing with the make up of a person's personality. They break down into the following areas:
   1) Id – First to develop, only interested in pleasure regardless of reality or conseqence. i.e. sexy movie, lets jerk off now!
   2) Ego – develops age three. Brings a reality focus behavior. i.e. sexy movie, I want to jerk off so I'll go into the can so I won't disturb anyone or get arrested.
   3) Superego – Gives a moral reality focus from our caregivers. i.e sexy movie, I'd like to jerk off, but that's wrong and may hurt society. So I'll hold off realizing that this delayed gratification will eventually pay off and I can have a sexually gratifying relationship.
3. Number of relationships. We have mentioned this before but the number and durations of a females past relationships is of great importance. How many relationships? How many co-habitations? Co-habitations are very closely related to marital relationships. How long was each of these serious relationships? Did she move in with a guy right away? That could indicate poor judgment or very impulsive behavior. Both of these would indicate intense study of this woman for issues. If she doesn't want to talk about these past relationships maybe she has something to hide? Look very deep.

THE MEDICINE CABINET

Yes we know that this is devious but all's fair in love and war. When at your new girlfriends house/apt, go to the bathroom and look in her medicine cabinet. If you see pills in there look at the names of the drugs. If there are several bottles you should write the names of the drugs down. She could be taking these medicines for a mental instability or a disease. Some of the more popular anti-depressants and psychoactive drugs are:

1) Prozac – Anti-depressant very popular
2) Celexa – New generation anti-depressant
3) Effexor – Old generation anti-depressant
4) Ativan – Anti-anxiety drug
5) Xanax – Very popular anti-anxiety drug.
6) Depakote – Used for treatment in Bi-polar/manic depressive
7) Seroquil – New Generation anti-psychotic
8) Haldol – Old generation anti-psychotic
9) Valium – Old generation anti-anxiety drug

Other medications to watch out for:

1) Acyclovir – Herpes treatment
2) Condylox – Herpes
3) Valtrex – New Herpes drug
4) Zivorax – Herpes
5) Fuzeon – New aids drug
6) Famciclovir – Aids
7) Retrovir – Aids
8) Combivir – Aids

Typically if you see anything with a 'vir" in the name check it out. It can be for any of the viral based diseases, (aids, hepatitis B, C or non B non C). Finding these drugs could very well save your financial and physical life.

There are many more, but when in doubt write them down. You can take them to the pharmacy or look them up on the Internet. Just note the number of the medicines she takes. An average 23 year old woman shouldn't have anything more that Aspirin, Tylenol, birth control pills, and vitamins. Women with mental or STD problems must come under the most intense scrutiny!!!!

Yes it's a shitty disguising thing to prejudge people by their medicine cabinet. Your prospective girl should have full disclosure before you fall in love with her, (or have sex with her). But if you don't know you could end up carrying home more than your luggage. Our purpose is to warn and inform. We have done so....

MENTAL STABILITY

Mental stability. When you're in a soul searching talk with the girl of your dreams, over a quiet drink, casually let the conversation drift into health. See what comes up from the conversation. Was she ever in rehab? The ha ha hotel? I've worked in the Psychiatric community for 4 years. Depression and women run hand in hand it seems. Attention Deficit Disorder is for the boys and Depression is for the girls. We don't know why, it just seems that way. During that time you wouldn't believe the number of extremely good looking women I came into contact with. They range from mildly depressed to manic-depressive, drug addictions to suicide attempts. You can't tell these women apart from the general population. If I met 70% of these women on the street I would have asked them out. Breathtaking as they were, they were crazy as a flock of Loons. Some of the types of mental instability are listed:

Depression. Hits a lot of women hard around 25-30 thirty years of age. You really don't do anything wrong, they're just unhappy with their lot in life. A chemical in-balance of the neuro-transmitters of the brain. The old days they called it melancholy. It can range from mild to acute even causing suicidal actions or tendencies. Beware of getting sucked into the "Vortex of the Victim". These women are needy and will suck you dry of their never ending desire for your attention, time and cash.

Suicide Queens. In severe cases of mental instability the chance of self–threatening/destructive behavior is high. Women sometimes say to their boyfriends or husbands "if you leave me I'll kill myself" or just after a severe fight she'll do a suicidal gesture, (act of committing suicide like a small cut on he wrists) to get your attention and/or your enslavement. The best counter for this type of action is recognition of the sub-species and book before you're involved too deeply. Once in it takes a lot to get out. One man had to leave the state without a forwarding address to escape the emotional terrorism of one suicide queen. Psychiatrists, psycho-active drugs and admissions to the crisis stabilization unit, (read the "Ha-Ha Hotel) all of the time will break your finances and your hopes for a happy life. Suicide queens use vortex behavior extensively. Beware!

Self-medication. Other women will take alcohol or drugs to "self medicate" their depression or mental instability. Always look at drinking to excess and drugs usage as a potential mental instability problem.

Either way, committing to a woman afflicted like this is a loadstone you don't want. These people typically don't get better with time. Depressed at 23 when she's at her best will probably be totally fucked up at 43. Do you need this ride? They'll throw you off your highway of success and into the back roads of obscurity and failure. Additionally if you continue on in the relationship there is a chance that she can pass her mental instability to YOUR children and you can watch with pride the self-destruction of your offspring through the rest of your life, (hint: mental illness is genetic).

Borderline personality. We feel that this is one of the most dangerous mental instabilities to have. The female borderline can be very functional, very charming, very sexy, and very manipulative especially with men. Sex can be so exciting it's breathless with these types of women. They can have a history of short, intense drama driven relationships with men/ women, (none of the failed relationships are viewed as the borderlines fault). They rarely take responsibility for their own actions and can mask their symptoms well. Once they feel the "safety" of a new partner in a relationship they will eventually start to expose their borderline side. Initially they worship and adore their partner. Then after a short while they shift to visualizing their partner as the source/blame of all of their problems. They fail to see their own contribution to the situation. They frequently project their issues on to the partner. Everything is black and white, right or wrong. They're highly intolerant of, or unable to adjust to the gray areas in life. They do well in fundamentalist type of religions because of the rigid "black and white" structure. They can make your life a living hell and then some. They tend to be highly abusive in relationships. Their relationships often collapse with rage, bitterness and total chaos once the partner is devalued in the females mind. This devaluation can take a couple of months to a couple of years to cycle through depending on the circumstances. This isn't a chemical imbalance per say, it's more of a dysfunction of the woman's personality by an outside force. Like a fucked up childhood, or some emotional trauma.

War Story. Monica and Carl fell in love. When they first met the relationship was breathtaking. Monica viewed Carl as the "morning and evening star" in her life. She hand one hand on the frying pan and the other on his pecker telling him how much she loved him. They were married and had a child. About 2 years after the marriage she started telling Carl "HE'S" changed. For months they argued about his change. When it finally was sorted out Carl hadn't changed, Monica had. After Carl was "devalued" in her mind, the hands came off the frying pan and the pecker, (they had sex about once a year weither Carl needed it or not). Through many attempts at counseling, Carl could never get Monica to give him the love she initially gave. She became verbally and physically abusive. Every day had drama in it. The marriage finally ended when Carl asked her "What is it that I do that pisses you off so much"? She replied "I don't know, you just do, matter of fact I can't stand you or even be in the same room as you". This was four years ago and to this day Carl still doesn't know what he did to piss her off.

War Story. Linda was an officer in the Army. During the second Gulf War she was assigned to our unit. Women have a distinct advantage in the military secondary to the lopsided male to female ratio. The power of her "camel toe" is amplified 10X in theater. During an activation of one year, she had no less than eight confirmed relationships, (despite the fact that she was engaged to another officer back in the states). We're not just talking sport fucking here. She was seriously "in" a relationship with these men. They all started off intensely powerful. This is the one, I'm so in love… etc but all of them ended in calamity and drama. She kept all of her men on the edge all of the time. Fights broke out, and at one point she tried to run down a Captain with her vehicle because he wanted to break it off with her. To avoid a court-marshal she eventually got sent home early to "quiet the unit down".

The borderline should be avoided at all costs. As we see from the war stories it can take a couple of years to "see" the true person you've married. This is why we advocate the three years of marriage before children policy. Eventually the pathological female will let her guard down and you can see the true "beast". Then you can make the decision to procreate, (have kids).

Manic Depressive. This is another dangerous personality trait for women. The affliction is a chemical imbalance that causes severe highs and lows in people. When the person is high their high is fantastic and when they come down the low is so debilitating they do destructive behaviors up to and including suicide.

War Story. One female I counseled had been stable on her prescriptions for eight years. She had a very good, job, a child and was well respected. Then one day for no apparent reason flipped out. Her body chemistry might have changed and her drugs were no longer able to balance her mind. One day she took her credit cards and in one week charged thirty thousand dollars shopping. She spent the week partying leaving her 7year old son alone at home. Her manic period finally ended when she had a three-some with her friend and her husband. Then she crashed sinking into the depressive side of the mental state. Feeling she had to repent for her actions, she slashed both of her forearms from the wrist to her elbow.

While I was counseling her, she started out depressed and remorseful, then she "cycled", (meaning she switched to her manic or "up" side) and even though I was married at the time, she said "You're cute would you like to fuck"? How would you like to be married to this woman? She eventually got balanced on her medicine and got back to her life and the payment of the $30,000 in credit card debt she had accumulated. The frightening fact is that this woman was extremely attractive. She was dressed exceptionally well, articulate and sophisticated. Virtually any single man, (including myself) seeing this woman on the street would jump to ask her out. Her "secret" would probably be brought out when lots of great sex and when love was established in the relationship. "Vortex" behavior would most likely be used here.

These aren't all of the mental problems that people experience, but these are some of the pitfalls that men can fall into when saddled with a woman who is mentally unstable. Look for the clues now rather than later when you have already brought the cow.

THE DISCLOSURE

Since we're talking about finding problems we must now talk about disclosure. When a woman meets a man she doesn't at first say, "Hi, I'm a manic depressive"! Or "Hi I have a sex addiction and have problems with remaining faithful". No they'll usually play the game of the "nice" girl. She'll describe herself as a good girl who has done the right thing only to be a victim to an unscrupulous fuck stick, (the last guy she dated /lived with/married). They can keep this game up for a very long time for women are very good at "games". Matter of fact they may even believe it because they're in denial, (see denial chapter 3). What you have to do is determine what is truth and what isn't.

1) When talking to your babe, try to get several versions of her sad victim story. Keep them in your mind as far as content and sequence. Then at some later date ask her again about Mr. Fuck-stick. Does the story follow the same general idea or does it tend to drift regarding her facts. If she's drifting then that's a sign to look a little deeper into her past relationships and issues.
2) Go out with her friends. This is typically very hard to get men to do. Make this a point that you want to "do" things with her, to include her friends. If she balks about going out with her friends. That's a warning sign she might have something to hide. When out with her friends watch the interaction of her with the girls. What are they talking about'? What kind of moral background do her friends have? If a woman has a lot of whore friends then she might be one herself. One whore friend in a group is usually okay. Everybody has at least one friend that's labeled a whore. Even though these are her friends they still "snipe" at each other.

Snipes are little digs at each other that can add direction to your covert investigation.

3) How do her friends see her? What could be dangerous is if her friends see her as the "whore" of the group! These people have known her for some time and probably have seen her when she doesn't have the facade up.
   There are two things you should find out: (1) How long has she been in this group, and (2) What do her friends think of her as a friend, a confident and a human being?
4) The angry or jealous friend. When out with her friends there might be an "angry or jealous friend". Angry or jealous friends aren't really friends at all but they hang out with different groups for number safety in bars. Or just that they're so dysfunctional they can't get along with anybody and glom onto whatever group that'll tolerate them. The angry or jealous friend can be a wealth of information. Remember though never act on the angry or jealous friend's information solely. Confirmation of this information is essential because of the agenda of the angry or jealous person might be to break up your relationship.
5) The Relationship Resume - Old boyfriends. This isn't as easy to get reliable information about. The old boyfriend can be a wealth of information. Information about him will unfortunately have to be indirectly obtained. Old boyfriends usually don't talk to the new guy fucking his squeeze, (especially if she broke it off with him). Your best bet is to get the old ones' names and look at their reputation if possible. Boyfriend #1 had no job and rides motorcycles all day long. She had to take care of him. Boyfriend #2 was in a band. She had to take care of him. Boyfriend #3 had no career working a series of odd jobs. She still had to take care of him. With a boyfriend resume like this you have to look very hard to your girlfriend's mental state. Maybe she likes the "bad boys" and is a storm-damaged boat in need of a harbor? Or maybe she's just shit stupid and will fall for any ridiculous offer? Regardless of why, do you want this woman to raise your child? Note: talk to her friends and try to get them started talking about her ex-.
6) Look at her family. Like with the friends look for the interaction between Mom and Daughter. Strained, distant angry or confrontational? How does Mom relate to dad? The existence of issues can be determined here. When you see some irregularities here, question her later. Questioning when she has had a few drinks is good. Liquor tends to "loosen the tongue". How she

relates to her mother or father could be how she'll relate to her child, (or to you).

7) Mistakes. Everyone can make mistakes in life, (even men). The big question is if the female has made a mistake, has she learned from it? In the boyfriend resume above apparently the female has demonstrated a pattern for acquiring worthless men. You have to ask yourself "why"? One fuck-stick at a young age is acceptable, three or four of them is a pattern of mistakes you don't want to own. Some things you might want to examine is:
    a. Constant bad boys. As we said above this can be a "storm damaged boat". Or it can be a desire for the wild life. Either way it warrants intense investigation.
    b. Abortions. One can be dealt with. Two or more show a pattern of shit stupid actions. If you got pregnant once you might fucking figure out what caused it and take some sort of protection against it.
    c. Financial insolvency/mismanagement. This is a good indicator of organization. Is she living from paycheck to paycheck? Does she have a budget? Does she plan? If she doesn't then you'll have to live with her financial fuck-ups. This will, of course, be with your money as well. Once married you are financially responsible for her financial insolvency and fuck-ups as she is yours.

War Story. Lynn was married to Mike. He used to abuse her until she eventually got tired of his shit and called the police. The fuck-stick got arrested for abuse. He had no job and when he tried to get a public defender Lynn discovered that he couldn't. He was married to her and since she had a job and was his wife she had to pay for his attorney to get him off the hook.

    d. How did she "solve" her problems. How she solved past problems will be most likely how she'll solve future problems with you.
        i. Is she a runaway? Does she have a tendency not to face up to reality and scoot? Sucks to be you if you're married with children.
        ii. Did she look for a "savior" to rescue her? Again if you're married, have children and have trouble will she look for a rescuer to save her, (read fuck a guy at work and want him to take her away from it all).
        iii. Does she just sit and flounder in her misery? This is very common. Women can sit and simply do nothing

to end the shit soup they're in. Not attractive choice either.

iv. Does she dig her heels in and work to solve her problem? This, of course, is the right answer. Even if she's not the sharpest knife in the drawer mentally, it demonstrates that she has a good attitude you can work with. (follow up question: does she know when the battle has been lost and it's time to retreat to regroup?)

8) Internet investigation. For a relatively small fee, ($10.00-$100.00) you can check out a person with regards to criminal offenses, bankruptcy, child abuse, bad checks and a myriad of other things. $100.00 is a small amount compared to 15 years of child support or ½ of your savings and house.
9) Private investigator. It sounds like so much spy shit, but if you got the money you would be surprised at what you can find out about a person through a PI. A good PI has sources for really good background searches. Think about it. The government does background checks on people for their important jobs. Why shouldn't you do a background check on the mother of your children? Cost is high here, but if you marry and divorce making $50,000 a year you could end up paying $120,000 – 180,000 for child support over twenty years. Now add in ½ of your savings, house equity and retirement. A PI investigation is cheap relatively speaking.

Regardless of these actions the best path is to take it slow. Time will usually tell all. Don't gloss over the warning signs no matter how good the pussy is. Most women can't hide serious personality/mental defects forever. Remember the three year policy for having children. Given enough time flaws will usually surface and you can decide to act without too much financial and emotional cost.

FINANCIAL WORTHYNESS (CHAMPAGNE TASTE… BEER BUDGET)

As we said above once committed/married the female will undoubtedly have access to your bank account. This will be either in the direct or indirect sense. Examination of her spending habits should be a discriminator for your mate selection. If you you're fucking filthy rich and don't give a damn about money you can skip this section. If not, you'd better pay attention.

Look at your female generally. How is she dressed? What are her tastes? Does she drive a fancy car? Does she yearn for a Range Rover? Is this demand for expensive shit balanced with her financial ability to pay for it? If not then if you're going to be married to her YOU will be the expediter of her dreams and wants.

Also as mentioned above does she pay he bills on time? Does she take her financial commitments seriously? Are bills late? Does she get calls from creditors? All of this paints a picture of the woman you'll be financially tied to.

Actions on the objective.

1. Look at her mail. Look at the number of her bills due and from where. Lots of fashion stores bills are a bad sign. Look for bills in red envelopes or printed on red paper. These typically indicate a serious past due status.
2. Examine her spending vs. income ratio. Add up the approximate value of her "things" and equate it to her income. If it's really lopsided ask yourself the question "How does she pay for all of this shit"?
4. Consumption patterns. Does she "squander" all of her money? Does she "can't wait for payday". Warning sign: if she has to borrow from you to make a bill stand back and look real hard. Even though she pays you back, this can indicate poor financial planning. Does she have to "re-buy" lots of shit because she doesn't take care of her stuff?
5. Go shopping. Yes I know that this is commensurate to a death sentence, but necessary. It will also get you points for being a good sensitive guy. Watch her buy clothes. Does she look for the sales? Is she in love with designer/name brand shit?
6. Credit report. This is the best way to determine her status. Getting it will be tricky though. One way is announce that you hand her should buy a house. That you need a credit report to establish your combined loan potential. The internet has several places to get this information easily and cheap.

This issue can be a major deal breaker or a slight speed bump in the road depending on your personal circumstances. Again we advocate looking at the total female package and weighing this information before final commitment takes place.

SMOKING

Although we've talked about this earlier it warrants reinforcing. Smoking is often glossed over secondary to love and sexual issues. When this subject comes up the woman frequently feels that, "If you love me then love me as I am". This sounds so wonderful if you're reading one of those cheap paperback chic novels. But once we get back to the real world it's quite different. If you're a smoker fine you two can puff along until your lungs give out. If you're not then this is important criteria to consider. If she's smoking other than socially when you broach this subject and explain this is a deal breaker she might offer to quit.

I'LL QUIT FOR YOU BABY.....maybe

Typically when a woman quits smoking for the sake of a man she doesn't really quit, (permanently). When the first drink flows smoking is typically like air to them. They crave it like we crave sex. Cigarettes are very addictive for women and the likely hood of a long term cessation is not likely. The most likely scenario is she quits until you're married and will probably start up after some significant emotional event of her choosing. Make your decision now and either drop the smokestack or keep her. If she does stay quit then consider yourself lucky. Very few people are able to quit and stay quit.

Let's say you make it to retirement with a smoker. Many smokers develop Congestive Obstructive Pulmonary Disease, (COPD). This results in diminished physical capacity, (read invalid) and having her tote around an oxygen tank all the fucking time? Think about kissing those lips with that snotty oxygen tube hanging out of her nose, Mmmm... I get excited just thinking about that don't you? Maybe take a walk down a beach for a whole 12 feet before she turns blue and passes out from the effort. How can you make love to her when she doesn't have the wind to hump back. Happy retirement, sucks to be you. Taking care of a smoker is also expensive. Smokes are expensive, (price out a pack a day x 365 x 20 years and see what you get). When they get older and are all fucked up from the smokes the hospital bills, the oxygen tanks and all those drugs to keep her ass alive the costs can bury you. Think hard about falling in love with a smoker.

BE ALL THAT YOU CAN BE

One important note that we feel you should consider when selecting your partner. This is the absolutely best that she'll be in your relationship. Typically she's on her best behavior and full of love for you. Your the romance she's always dreamed about. Try to view her twenty years later. Will you be satisfied with her then? Any faults will only get larger with the passage of time. That's why we preach moderation in selecting a woman. We emphasize to look at the aggregate (total or whole) woman before you make your selection.

ALL'S FAIR IN LOVE AND WAR

To recap, this chapter it is to allow the man to visualize "his" perfect woman, (you won't meet "her" but you'll be close). This process will place this mental picture in your mind and allow you to focus on the type of woman you need to accomplish your goals in life.

We know you have to be in love have reasonable sex and all that. But as we said earlier, you can fall in love with a decent, educated and caring woman who will be your partner who will be supportive and grow old with you. Or you can fall in love with a whore who will fuck you in your bed, fucks you in the head, fucks your buddy instead and then fucks you in court when she dumps your ass sending you into the "pit of financial despair". If you don't date whores then your chances of loving one is slim. If you set your standards high and date only the suitable ones, (who match your profile) then your chances are reasonably good you'll find and love the "right girl".

We might be a little intense when it comes to "checking out" your female. It might even be a little overboard, and cash intensive. But all's fair in love and war as is all's fair in hate and divorce. If the cash is great enough she won't hesitate for a moment to have private investigators look up your asshole to find some dirt for court. She'll rake your ass over the coals in court and have no problems sleeping like a baby the same night. If you consider what you can loose from a divorce w/children the cost/ time spent is relatively very small. Is what we suggested fair? No but President Jack Kennedy said it best, "Life isn't fair". YOU have to protect your future children. YOU have to protect your finances. YOU have to protect your personal future. If you fail to heed our warnings then you'll increase your chances of hooking up with the "wrong girl". Forewarned is forearmed, you have the knowledge to select the right mate. Don't waste your time, your money and your life on the wrong one. Remember "Every date is a possible mate".

CHAPTER 7

THE DATING GAME

Now that you have developed a profile of the type of woman you would consider the "perfect" mate, you may now date in an "informed" status. As we said earlier you don't run around bars, social functions or any other place with a copy of your profile, (unless you're socially challenged). Note: Never talk about it or allow the female to see your profile. This would put you in the "shit stupid" category. Again this is an "in-house" document. The whole profile exercise was developed to help YOU "mentally" focus in on what YOU want vs. what you NEED to be successful in your life and your timeline.

Understand there is no "Miss Right", Miss 100% solution or "Miss Perfect". There is however a "Miss Real Close To" and "Miss 72%" solution though. Don't set your goals of finding a 100% solution of your profile in a woman. That's why we had you prioritize your desires. Try to focus your efforts on the high priority traits, (>7/10).

FINDING "THE" GIRL

Where do you find the "perfect" mate? First take a mental look at your profile. What's high on the list for you? If it's a hot body built for sin and fucks like a banshee then you simply hang out at those spots. Bring your checkbook though. These girls don't come cheap and usually have an insatiable lust for money. They work real hard getting ready to play real hard. They know they're hot, and will undoubtedly look for the best deal.

The smart ones will play hard until they start to see their youth fade. Then they'll target a likely suspect and "settle down" to the calmer life, (at least until they get a couple of kids).

War Story. I had worked with an absolutely gorgeous woman named Ally. Her given name wasn't that but she changed it because Ally sounded much more sheik. She had worked very hard and long to get into nursing. She wasn't a natural nurse, and she really didn't seem that interested in nursing. But her lack of successes in nursing didn't bother her too much. She was focused on her real goal. Her sole reason to go to nursing school and get into the ICU was to meet a Doctor, preferably a surgeon. She pointed this out to us several times, (she had a profile established as well). For two years she would trash out good men only to wait for the doctor she wanted. She eventually left our hospital because the doctors were all too old; really they were just wise to the situation and her. They had been married to "Ally" types and some were divorced as well. She did her research and found out that all the "interns", (young "uninformed" doctors) were at the teaching hospitals. She was cold, calculating and eventually did achieve her goals getting pregnant by one of the surgical residents in the Medical Center. Will she get divorced? I guess time will tell. She's a bought woman who used sex and pregnancy to attract and marry her target. This isn't a recipe for a long-term marriage. But this is what happened, and you'll see this time and time again. Only the situation and names will be different. Pretty girl, successful guy as Tina Turner said, "What's love got to do with it?"

BIRDS OF A FEATHER FLOCK TOGETHER

So where does a good guy find the good girl? If you look back to older times you will see schools like Wellesley, Vassar and Smith colleges. Why were these schools developed? Typically women went from daddy to husband, or daddy to college to husband. This was a time where all that women really needed to know was how to please the man and raise children. Why the tremendous expenditure on a woman's education? It's simple. The wealthy fathers of these girls wanted their little girls to meet someone nice and respectable. They also were wise to educate the girls to make suitable companions for the men. These schools were the female compliment of the "Ivy" league male schools. They would interface in social events with the men's colleges. The well to do women would meet with the well to do men and the right kind of husbands would be procured, (for proper breeding of course). The general rule of propinquity was in place; if you have your daughter only hang around with well to do guys from good families she'll probably meet, date, fall in love, and marry a well to do guy from a good family. Now that didn't guarantee your daughter would come home with an Ivy League all around good guy, (the Ivy League had fuck sticks too). Not as many as in the general population but they were there. Your daughter could also come home with the janitor but this was very rare. All in all the percentage of good mates warranted the continued practice of this method. We do this today. Parents didn't want you "hanging out" with the "wrong crowd". If you did you would eventually end up in trouble. Most parents want their children to go to a good school to get a good education and meet a "nice girl". You'll undoubtedly want your children to go to a nice place to meet a good mate. I mean do you really want "your" daughter to marry some low rent fuck stick that will probably fuck up her college, career, leave her maybe pregnant, (or with several kids) and eventually dump them on your door step to raise? Unless you're shit stupid then you probably won't. It's simply the human element in action. We want you to equate this to your own mating practices.

So how does this apply to your search for a mate? "If you lie with dogs you're probably going to get fleas". If you hang with whores all the time the chances are you'll probably fall in love with one. Typically these women are very manipulative and are able to convince a guy of anything, (especially if vortex behavior is used). So where do you go? Find places where the women believe in the same things you believe in. Women who understand responsibility, hard work and has some moral upbringing. Try looking in the business world, institutions of higher education, or church. Don't make the bar the only place you hang out to look for women. This is fine for sport fucking, but not the best place to find a quality woman.

WOMEN AT WORK

We said to look for women in the business world. But we recommend that you not look for them at your immediate place of business. This is a too close for comfort situation, (It is okay to "graze" in other departments though).

Example: You work for Acme Inc. You are the junior accountant in purchasing. Dating a marketing analyst in overseas sales is acceptable. Dating the other junior accountant in purchasing is not recommended.

Never date a woman directly associated with your work. This basically means YOUR office, suppliers, and people whom your progress in work is "directly" tied to the good relations of this person. Some reasons for NOT having a relationship in your office.

1) Subordinate love affairs. If she's subordinate to you her good or poor work performance will be attributed to your relationship or break-up of your relationship. She won't get a fair deal and neither will you. If you're going to leave the job, okay, but anything else don't.
2) POSTULATE #6 FEMALES WILL ALWAYS TALK TO SOMEONE. Women have this innate desire to talk out their problems. The majority of women develop friendships at work, (even if that's not "business smart" thing to do). Since they don't have the "community of sisters" in their neighborhoods they establish a benign sisterhood at work. Any problems you have with her will be broadcast all over the work place. Chances are she will eventually spill her guts to her friend about her "woes". You're now a fuck stick of a lesser order. In business you want a clear demarcation, (line in the sand) between your personal life vs. your professional life. Because the fact that you like to sit in front of the TV and pick your nose and scratch your nuts shouldn't be known by anybody except your significant other. Women will talk.
3) You can also get into competition with her professionally. We can't think of a more rewarding, bonding and couple oriented experience than having your girlfriend get your promotion, (your buddies will really support you while their thumping your nuts severely).
4) Breaking up. Remember POSTULATE #1 SHE WILL FORGIVE, BUT NEVER FORGET. If you wrong her no matter how honorable and professional you were in the relationship you will be the fuck stick of the year to all she comes in contact with. If she holds the purse strings to your sales, funding for projects or whatever you can be potentially screwed. Also in business no one can afford bad press. Having her tell all her friends how you fucked her over when things were going so well. It doesn't matter she had the temper of Attila the Hun. Her friends will never know that part of the relationship. Note: she could tell all the women, (and men) how much of a ridiculous fucking joke you are in bed, (which we know is so untrue). But why waste your efforts performing damage control when you could be making progress at work or having fun.

War Story. Tim was a fellow reserve officer. Good man decent and very much into doing the right thing. He started dating a coworker. Eventually the relationship blossomed into cohabitation for over two years. During this time he found out that she wasn't the one for him. They had issues regarding her temper and some religion problems. So he openly expressed his feelings and his decision, (after six months of couples counseling) to break up. She accepted his decision but when he went to work the females on the staff were cold to him. Regardless of how nice he was when he broke up, how nice of a guy he was at the office, he was now the company fuck stick. The feelings from her female friends eventually spilled over to the men and he was in a very unpopular position. He eventually left the company expressly because of the above situation. He wasn't planning to leave, but he had to in order to escape the bad PR he was encountering.

Actions on the objective. Look for women who fit into your profile. You're not a snob you're just focused. Stay away from the office related romance. If you find yourself in a romance with a co-worker either quit the job or the girl. Business is business and love is love. The two should never meet. EVER!

ALPHA LEADERSHIP

The goal of our book isn't how to date. We just want to show you how to avoid some of the pitfalls associated with unfocused dating. The most important aspect of the dating sequence is the establishment of the alpha dog, (or alpha leader/man). This is simply the dominant personality in the relationship. In all relationships weather it's man and wife or two dogs in a cage. Someone will have to be the alpha leader. If you think that a relationship is really governed on a 50/50 basis then you need to quit watching the women's channel on television. It is imperative that you be the man/alpha leader, (duh). Fail this and the female will forever control you. You will be treated like a child, asking for permission to do things, having her lord over you for whatever you want to do. If that's the way you want it then fine. Stop reading our book and give it to a real man you pussy!

Responsibilities of alpha leadership. Attaining the alpha leadership also carries great responsibilities. Responsibilities are:

1) You can't sit in the cheap seats and thump the ref's nuts. You're the leader and if you fail in this you'll be the responsible party.
2) No Rogue Dictators. The alpha leader can't be a despot or a dictator. Being the boss requires benevolence, wisdom, justice and self-restraint. That means you don't drop her date night just to go out with the buds. Tyrants get over thrown, and you would be left wondering what happened.

3) Chief planner. You're responsible for the planning of the family. This includes the finances, the retirement and all matters of importance. If you fuck it up you're at fault. Always remember though only a fool would not include your spouse in this planning. Let her know her input is wanted and critical for the decision process. But you're the final word on the plans.
4) If you're a pussy and let her do all the planning and leading if she fails you're still going to be responsible for the fuck-up.

ESTABLISHMENT OF THE ALPHA LEADER

Establishment of the alpha leader should be easy for the man who has a clear idea of where he's going in life. His mission statement and time line, (see Appendix A) give him a purpose and a path to follow. Because of this he's confident of himself and his abilities. If a man has confidence it will pore over into the relationship and the woman will pick up on this quickly. Actually she'll be attracted to this confident attitude. Your confidence will pave the way to becoming the alpha leader.

Resistance of alpha leader. Some women fight you being the alpha leader. Now what do you do if the woman doesn't allow you to be the alpha leader? Some of the reasons she might not allow you to be the Alpha leader:

1) You're a pussy. Yes that's the case sometimes. The first step is to look into your-self. Are you acting like a man, being a leader? Do you have a plan? Are you focused? Or are you simply floating around in the ocean like a piece of fucking drift wood waiting for a woman to "complete" you, (read: another Mommy to take care of you)?
2) Trust Issues. Woman who can't allow the man to be the alpha dog could have severe trust issues. Did something happen in her childhood, high school, and college? Did Daddy leave her, did Mommy? This is an indication to dig deeper into her background.
3) Male-female switching. In "Men are From Mars, Women are From Venus", Dr. Gray explains that for women to compete successfully in the workplace they tend to switch to their "male side" while at work. That is they act like men when at work. Does she have trouble switching back over to her feminine side when she's with you? Maybe she likes it when she's in her male side? If her need to be the alpha leader is severe then it's decision time. You might want to cut the rope before she drags you in.

BIBLICAL MANDATE FOR ALPHA LEADERSHIP

Male alpha leadership is even supported by the Bible. 1 Peter Chapter 3 verse 20 says: Wives submit! For ye are the weaker vessel. Sounds pretty good huh? However if you read on you will find that Peter also said: Husbands cherish your wives as Christ cherished the church. What you have here is the owner's manual for life. It's clearly the man's job to rule, but he also needs to hold dear his subjects. Be fair, be wise and don't abuse your role as the natural God given leader of the woman.

Note this is a religious "silver bullet". It only works on devout Christian women. It's very tricky to use in debate. Tell this to the average female she'll look at you like you've lost your mind.

Actions on the objective. Remember; the man is the natural leader. Establish the alpha leader immediately in the relationship. Normal women should not have a problem with this. Departures from normal are dangerous and need to be looked at closely. If you can't establish the alpha leadership then continue to date in an "uncommitted" status or split up. Resistance in the woman won't get any better with the passage of time.

THE INITIAL DATING PERIOD

There are many dangers during the initial dating period? If you have established yourself as the alpha dog then you are ahead of the power curve. But even though you have this position doesn't mean there won't be challenges to your title. This is a normal function of the female but even if this is normal it doesn't mean you shouldn't prepare for it. You could still loose it if you're sloppy. After successfully holding and practicing good alpha leadership for a while she'll begin to trust you and challenges to your leadership should be less.

Alpha Dog skirmishes. Some women will "test the waters" of the male leadership. Attacks to your alpha leadership start with little skirmishes. A skirmish is a small battle designed to wear you down, examine your political will power, test you or the relationship. You're in a relationship cold war of attrition. It might be the change of an agreement for dinner, weekend activity or something that isn't openly important to you. Recognition of the situation is paramount. You don't have to mount a war. Dealing with this is like dealing with a child. Be consistent and softly firm but the operative word is firm. If she makes a deal with you it's a deal. Departures from the agreement for poor reasons are not allowed no matter how small it is. If she displays a valid reason for changing a plan then agree to it if you can. "Because I want to" or "because I don't like it" are not valid reasons. This is how you train the female. Pouting, anger, crying and with holding sex doesn't go here. Oh yeah sex can't work here either, (see section on arguing and the power of the pussy). Don't let her sway you with lust, hold firm, (no pun intended).

EMOTIONAL INACCESSIBILITY

We're not writing a "How to" book on dating. But we do want to detail one important relationship concept that we believe supports maintenance of Alpha leadership. That is the concept of being "inaccessible". When you're in a relationship it's important not to be too "accessible" to your partner. If you do then your partner will get bored with you and take advantage of you. This shouldn't be confused with hiding or being secretive. You must be available and unavailable at the same time. It's a difficult task to master but once you do then alpha leadership is easy.

The alpha leader has a purpose. He is aloof, he has a mission and a plan. He carries a mystic quality about himself. He's the "Old Spice Guy" or "The Marlborough Man". Believe it or not we've found out that many women are terribly attracted to this concept. She feels that she has you but she still questions if she really has you. When your woman can say she feels that she knows everything about you, but also knows that it's only what you want her to know, you've achieved emotional inaccessibility.

War Story. Greg was with Deborah and suffering badly. Greg was very athletic and out going while Deborah would sit at home all of the fucking time doing nothing, smoke cigarettes, and bitch about everything that Greg did, (or didn't do). Sex with her was poor to shitty and was done on a "duty type" basis, (usually it took some arguing to get her to give it up). Greg was going insane with this situation. He always thought that if he "filled in the numbers of her paint by number dream" she'd fill in his. WRONG! This was painfully not the case. I explained "inaccessibly" to Greg and suggested that he become more inaccessible to Deborah. Greg said "fuck it" and started to go places and do things and not give a shit what Deborah thought or did. He reenacted his own plan, started following it and started to enjoy his life! He was always available to Deborah, but unavailable. She could always call him on the cell phone, but he was off... doing whatever he wanted to do, (kayaking, sailing or out with his friends). After a couple of months Deborah picked up on his emotional inaccessibility and made a 180 degree change. She started to make herself more "available" to Greg. She was following Greg's plan and they started to do more things together. She was more active, (joined a gym), and sex was approaching top shelf levels. She was taking Greg's lead and both were enjoying it. Note: Although Deborah was following Greg's plans, Greg was still sensitive to "her needs" but it was clearly Greg's decision to do so.

INTERMEDIATE DATING PERIOD

"Your girl" and you should be comfortable with each other. The sex should be top shelf and both of you should be having the best times of your lives. As the female becomes more secure in your feelings for her she will naturally "spread her wings" and test the boundaries of the relationship. The most important defining moment of the intermediate dating period is the "declaration of love". Unlike the Declaration of Independence, this document will foster commitment and induce an eventual partnership. It is imperative that the man set the relationship tempo here. Remember the old saying: "All roads lead to Rome". To a good woman, "All dating leads to love and eventually marriage". The Alpha dog should always be cognizant of this.

The love zone. Eventually thorough the course of the relationship it will become evident that you must enter the "L" zone. This is the proclamation of love. If you're not in love with the girl then you must make it perfectly clear that it isn't going anywhere for you, (or her). You should also stay away from any statements regarding her that has the word "love" in it. "I love being with you", I love your cooking or I love having sex with you" is a fuck-stick action. To a woman the utterance of their most holy word in any context can be easily confused.

"I love you" can mean many things depending on which sex said it and who said it first. For men it can mean, "yeah I love you", an expression of extreme like. For the woman it can be a covenant, sacred and eternal. When you're in a real "oh shit" relationship the mention of love must be thought out and planned. It would best for the man to say it first. Gain the moral high ground and support your leadership of the relationship. Remember you're the man, you're the leader. You set the tempo. So you must be prepared for this eventuality and have a prepared response to it. Remember Postulate #1, SHE WILL FORGIVE, BUT NEVER FORGET. Her happy remembrance of the first "I love you" will get you out of many scrapes later on. The love statement can happen several ways.

1) During a passionate interlude, (fucking for us working types). The female will work us into a sexual feeding frenzy and at the right time blurt out "I LOVE YOU"! You're into the great sex thing and might have a response that could be total reflex and respond in kind. Yes you said it but her objective was to get you to

say it. To get you familiar with the word and relaxed in saying it. Like a horse being broke, you place honey on the bit. The horse will like the honey and allow the bit to be placed in the mouth. Eventually the honey goes away, but the bit is there to stay. Note: Don't try and say the "L" word during sex your self. She won't take it seriously and it will probably piss her off or scare her off. After the "L" word has been said, then it's okay and preferable to say it during sex, (especially at the end of sex – see chapter on intimacy).

2) You're in a romantic spot. She looks in your eyes and says: "I love you". Now you are trapped. You have nothing to do; you can't claim the passions of sex made you do it. You have to deal with it in its entirety. Do you say it back? Only if you want to. But you must have a planed measured response. Always remember this is where the woman has bared her soul to you and her heart is in your hand, (or she's throwing the love bullet out there to give the relationship a little "nudge" in the right direction. Decision time again! If you don't tell her you love her it will send her self-esteem crashing down and if you stay with her, eventually marry her you will encounter POSTULATE #1, SHE WILL FORGIVE BUT NEVER FORGET. So when you're in the relationship update the status of your feelings for her on a regular basis. If you're in love, then say it. Don't be a pussy about it! If not in love then, and if you don't give a shit about her tell her you're having fun with her but haven't felt anything like that yet. If you know you're not going to make it with her love wise ever then do the right thing and cut her loose. She'll cry, won't eat for a few days and boo hoo to all of her friends but she'll get over it. Your honor isn't worth a piece of ass. Ass is too plentiful and too available.

3) The confrontation. After you date a girl for a while and nothing has been said yet regarding love she might confront you directly. She might say "we been dating for blah, blah, blah and I've been wanting to know just how you feel about me". A direct question requiring a direct answer. What has happened here is that you've just suffered a major attack on your alpha dog status? She's just had a counseling session with her as the superior and you as the subordinate. Now you're in between a rock and a hard place. You have to deal with the feelings issue, your lack of dealing with it first and her obvious frustration to your lackadaisical approach to the relationship. The interesting part here is that SHE hasn't said anything! She has no emotional investment at this point. You're

on a down hill lie, and the green is still a long fucking way off! Your choices are very limited. Tell her you don't know and will let her know when you do, (even if you do love her). Telling her you love her now is giving in to her setting the tempo of the relationship. It'll also encourage her to use this tactic more often since it got a "real good" response this time.

Regardless of what method you use, once committed to love your whole relationship changes. You now will enter the "we" zone of management, (see the covert commitment process). You have taken the first step to a permanent relationship.

THE FLIRT

This is a section that deals with an important aspect of female management. What to do when a women flirts? The flirt is considered anything provocative to the male in order to create enticement of a sexual nature. Let's look at that for a moment. Why would a woman flirt? Some of these are:

1) Specific flirtation. To gain the attention of a particular man. The woman wants to attract the attention of a guy she likes. She will be overly friendly, ask for his help, establish eye contact, smile at him, eat a Popsicle provocatively and a myriad of other things to garner his attention. This is considered normal. If she's lucky the man will respond, conversation will take place and so on and so on.
2) General flirtation. To gain attention of any or many men. This is a danger sign of the highest level. When woman generally flirt they have a hunger for attention that goes beyond companion or sexual desire. There isn't any particular mark, but it's like throwing chum, (blood and guts of fish to attract other fish) to attract anybody who will pay attention to her. We consider this non-normal and probably pathological with respect to our purposes. Women like this are attention seekers and don't warrant dealing with PERIOD! Attach yourself to one of these women and you'll either be in for a night of teasing, (or a lifetime of torture). They're long on having you pay attention to them and short on return. If they do consider you worthy of their affections it'll be a subservient relationship at best and when they tire of you, you'll be cast aside like so much human trash. STAY AWAY!!!
3) Flirting to make the guy jealous. This is another very dangerous manipulative behavior. You're dating a girl and you're not

paying what she feels is enough attention to her. So she garners some attention from some neighboring guy(s). Three courses of action:

a) Do nothing. Like any form of terrorism jealously flirting, (JF) should never be given into. Once you do then jealously will be the currency she'll use against you frequently. If she persists then our recommendation will be to dump her. She has placed her own wants/desires ahead of her concept of sanctity to a relationship.

b) Gestapo tactics. Go over and yank her ass back to you and get in a big fucking fight with her or the guy she's flirting with. Remember before getting into a fight with the guy. He's just trying to get laid. You can't beat up all the guys in the world she'll come into contact with. It's "her" actions you're mostly concerned about. Now if she's trying to get away from him and he won't let her then by all means beat the fucker's head in. She'll either be scarred or overjoyed that you did this. We don't recommend this. She'll be tempted to use this later.

c) Run over, pacify her and "make it right" for her. This is fine but we recommend that you use some lidocaine numbing jelly on the affected area before she puts in the nose ring. This is exactly the response she wanted and since it has been so successful she'll use it again, and again and again.

4) Once in a relationship and the woman hasn't displayed any flirtatious tendencies initially but suddenly does. What do you do? You have only two options on the initial incident.

   a. First set her down and explain the gravity of the situation. This must be done in a quiet controlled environment. Don't do it at the party or where the incident took place. Don't have sex with her until you have discussed the event either. Having sex prior to a bitch session ruins your position. Once you're discussing the event tell her what you saw, how you interpreted it and the seriousness of the situation. If she balks calmly tell her this isn't how you run your relationship. It's not how you are and if it happens again the relationship is over. The line is drawn in the sand. Explain that this is non-negotiable and will never be tolerated. This will also indicate a long intense investigation of her before commitment. If you're already committed then you need to take a step back in the relationship.

b. Trash the bitch now. If she has been really blatant you might not have a choice. Only you can judge the level of her flirting. If you think she can be salvaged then give her the "warning". Typically overt flirting doesn't get any better with the passage of time.

War story. This happened with me to a girl named Heidi. She flirted with a friend of mine. I gave her the "warning". Three months later she flirted with the same guy again. I told her the offense and the accountability of that offense. Despite her begging I stayed strong, (It helps to be pissed off at the time).

There's no room for a flirting woman. Don't live in denial on this! Look act, warn and act immediately if it happens again. Don't get caught in the weeds on this one. This is an ETHICS/ VALUES/ INTEGRITY (EVI) issue. EVI issues are non-negotiable issues. A woman either has it or she doesn't have it. Women who flirt are highly prone to cheat on their husbands/boyfriends. They crave the attention too much to stop and will eventually cheat on you.

ADULT RULES OF ENGAGEMENT

By this time the majority of all males have had at least one sexual experience. Most all males are or have been in some sexual relationship that involves regular contact with the female. Most all men and women have graduated from some sort of school and are out in the work force in some fashion or another. This phase involves the courtship of the female and then the eventuality of a long term relationship. Commitment vs. non-commitment.

Commitment... The word has a power all it's own. In the world commitment has the power to make even the poorest situation successful. In relationships it can be your helper or your hell. To women it is the holiest of feminine holy words. Like Yahweh, (the ancient word for God, only to be whispered once a year in the special temple by the high priest) it was and still is the holy grail of end states for the female. To men it's your completion, your competition or your condemnation depending on your choice of partners. The real trick is to know when you're being committed without your knowledge. This is called the "covert commitment process".

When in the dating mode and sex is usually being doled out in double helpings, men are very complacent. Relationships initially start out like a high from some illicit drug. You're making money, acquiring things, getting laid and are generally rich in the coin of the realm. In paraphrasing Ben Franklin, necessity is the mother of invention. Why did I say this? It's simple if you're getting your needs met, why do you want to change it? If it's not broke don't fix it... right? That's a good plan but it doesn't include the only wild card you have to hold. Yes, that's right, the female of the species. You may enjoy the ride so far, but if the girl isn't a slut, she will start the commitment process somewhere between six to ten months after penetration initially happens.

THE COVERT COMMITMENT PROCESS

The first steps into the covert commitment process will be acts of possession. You have seen these or have expected these many times in the past of your youth. What makes them different now is that the woman hears the faint "ticking" of her biological clock. She's opened the procreation window and likes the view. She now has an agenda, (like that's news). But this agenda isn't cut in stone, for she's at an impasse. She is faced with a life long choice: career vs. marriage/children. For the woman this is a defining moment and a critical point in your relationship lifespan.

You might not be aware of her decision process other than some slight moodiness. You might be given no choice in the matter, or maybe have some minor influence. But you'll undoubtedly share equally in any adverse consequences that erupt from her unilateral decision.

THE GOLDEN CARROT

You and your "babe" are doing all the things that you love her for, football games, sex, beer drinking on Fridays with your friends, sex, darts, sex, fishing, sex, hunting, sex, sailing, sex..... Get the picture? She's giving you a taste of her carrot. She's built a facade of what you consider the perfect mate. But in her mind you and the relationship has been mapped out for the future. She's used a combination of her dreams, fantasies and your reality to create this relationship and it's eventual outcome. Through the act of denial issues that she has concerning you have been purposely, selectively filtered out of her consciousness. She has already decided that what she doesn't like can be changed with feminine behavior modification, (see 'The Camel Toe Chronicles'). These issues will eventually be brought into the light at a later time and dealt with.

If things are too good to be true they usually are. So beware of the perfect mate. Mates are rarely perfect and if you find one step back momentarily and take time for a sanity check. We're not saying don't have a great time; enjoy the folly of love/lust. But be cognizant of the process that she is knowingly or unknowingly inflicting on you. Don't be angry with her either. She has a right to her agenda. Just as Canadian Geese fly south for the winter, women have commitment agendas. Even men have an agenda. We like to watch football games, have sex, go beer drinking with our friends, have sex, play darts, have sex, etc.... We all have agendas the woman naturally wants to activate hers.

Feminine Residue. Once out in the working world the woman can display possessiveness seen in less mature circumstances. This is considered normal for her in this stage of the relationship. However the first attack is usually an insidious one. You have your place, your job and your new car. Things are going great you met this girl and have been dating/fucking for around six to eight months. You have allowed the female to do sleepovers and have noticed that over the past few weeks she's been leaving "feminine residue". Feminine residue is the girly things that make life more comfortable for the female. They're divided into two categories. "General" residue and "specific or personal" residue. General residue can consist of but not limited to deodorant, tampons and maybe a douche. These are okay so long as they don't enter the "personal residue" category. Personal residue is anything that is owned individually by the female. Examples are toothbrushes, underwear, bras, and other personal items that are not generic in nature. The use of personal residue is her way of initially marking her territory and the first assault on your single status. This marking of her territory isn't just for other females. It's a symbolic saddle being placed on your back, not to strap it down and ride, but to familiarize you with it's feel and not be frightened with it. You are now presented with your first DEFINING MOMENT in the lifespan of your relationship and your alpha dog status. It 's what we call in the military recon by force. That is to attack a position in order to test the defenses and the political resolve of the objective, (notice that I didn't say enemy). What you do from this point on will undoubtedly affect your life to some degree. Some actions to this newly acquired residue could be:

1. Do nothing. This will send out a clear signal to the woman that you are okay with her residue and have tacitly given permission for her to "homestead" to a certain degree. Inaction on your part will invite a penetrating attack that we will describe later. Once this is allowed then you should consider taking the lead and defining the relationship and her status.

2. Gestapo tactics. Immediately insist that she immediately insist that she must package her residue up and remove it from the premises. This will of course answer the need to set limits as we discussed earlier. However it could and probably would have the adverse affect of terminating your relationship with her or at least turning her sexual performance commensurate an inflatable doll. Whatever the result it will not be pleasant for you. This is only done when you don't give a rat's ass about her or her feelings and self-worth/self-esteem.
3. Blame it on the roommate. This falls into the "chicken shit" category. You're not really being the man here but it does get the job done sometimes. Tell the female that your roommate is bitching about her staying here all the time and wants to divide up the rent by thirds instead of halves. This may or may not work, (unless you have an Einstein on your hands). It could also backfire if she says "great! I'll move the rest of my stuff in tomorrow. But if you're trying to keep the sex around and she's willing to believe it then give it a whirl. Note: only use this action if you have a roommate.
4. The "win-win" method. This is where you look for the "win, win" answer. One suggestion is to package her "personal residue" up immediately and bring it over to her place. Explain that you had noticed that she had forgotten her stuff and you were considerate enough to bring it on by. If you can time this with something special she really wants to do then all the better. With her in a hurry to go to whatever it was you had planned, it won't allow her to sit and dwell on this issue. There is a good chance you could escape immediate reprisal. Women will, if the man is rated high enough in her mind, want to believe that you had no conscious thought to your actions. They'll "take it in stride" and lay in wait for another opportunity to advance. This is an insurgency; it is a test of your political will.

PENETRATING ATTACK

It must be understood by the man that these actions are only delaying tactics at best. The eventually of the situation will be the placement of the "residue" either insidiously or openly in the dwelling of the man. What is the important thing here isn't weather you do or don't allow her residue in your place. It's that you understand the process at work and it's consequences. At this that time you can make an open and informed decision as to your future. Our recommendation is not to doddle. Remember you're the alpha dog, you set the tempo, not her. If you really care about her and have been dating successfully for a comfortable period then allow her openly to establish her presence there. Open talks before you allow this to happen to set the ground rules.

RELIGIOUS INCONGRITIES

As we stated in our profile chapter religious issues should have been weeded out during the first five dates. But since the profile is dynamic and changeable you have decided to date a woman who has a different religious background then you do. Always remember that this will always create some dissonance in your relationship. Since you have made the decision to "keep her" regardless of her religion then you have to completely shut the fuck up when she does it. You had your choice when you were dating.

BREAKING UP IS HARD TO DO

As the male travels through a relationship he has to understand that there is the potential that the woman he is dating isn't "the one" for him. Once he has realized this he must make the decision to break up. Many times in relationships the man has not broken up for a myriad of reasons:

1) It's not the right time, she is in school and it would devastate her life.
2) She's very vulnerable right now.
3) Her job is on the rocks.
4) She's had a family member die recently.

The list can go on and on and never end. Typically the real problem is that the man is a PUSSY! Yes that's right a pussy! It's in our nature to be the defender of the weaker sex. We're protectors, not some fuck-stick that breaks the poor female's heart. We don't naturally want to do this so we think up many reasons for to put it off. You have to be strong here. It might mean that you're going to a pseudo fuck-stick by calling it quits. If you stay with her because you're too much of a pussy to hurt her you can end up with the following:

1) You spend a large amount of time with her in a bad relationship wasting your youth and hers.
2) You get her knocked up and you're stuck like a Christmas pig.
3) She catches on to your pity of her and will use it to keep you, (and control you).

DO I LOVE OR DON"T I LOVE, (that is the question)

Now our book has detailed the women we want you to avoid when involved in a long-term relationship. If you have one of these undesirable women and you're fortunate enough to identify them it becomes pretty easy to do what should be done. If that happens then we feel good about writing this book.

Occasionally though you find a decent, caring and loving woman who is what we would consider the "right girl". The type we feel you should develop a relationship for. However the one little fact that we left out is "Do you love her"? Yes, sometimes even if it's the "right girl" you don't love her. No matter what you do it's not going to happen. Duke Ellington said it best, "It don't mean a thing if it ain't got that swing". So you have to do the "deed".

Like the alcoholic the first step to redemption is identification of the problem. If you followed our book then identification of the undesirable is easy. The "right girl" but you don't love her isn't. This is a much tougher nut to crack. But eventually you'll figure it out. And you eventually HAVE to do it. You're the leader even in the break up.

THE BAD GIRL DUMP

Breaking up with an undesirable woman is easy. You just say, "get the fuck out bitch", (or words to that effect). Keep it simple, direct and final. Don't give her a moment's notice to be manipulative or to plead, (or to offer great sex). Get pissed off at her if it helps. But don't be a pussy here!

THE GOOD GIRL BREAKUP

When having an unfortunate duty to perform it's best to get that duty over as quickly an as humanly as possible. Your message should be outlined and rehearsed. Give her the BLUF, (Bottom Line Up Front). Tell her your reasons for the breakup and DON"T discuss them with her. You can do that telephonically if she needs more closure. You must be gentle and firm, (the operative word is firm here). You try to be kind and decent but remember you have an unpleasant job to do.

Note: Once you've come to your decision don't run up and tell her with all of her friends and/or family. Arrange a meeting with her and tell her face-to-face. Don't ever tell her you're breaking up wither by mail or by telephone. There's no honor in doing that.

GRIEVING STAGES OF THE BREAKUP

We believe that the act of breaking up with someone (especially a woman) is like experiencing a death. A person can experience all, part or none of the stages of a death depending on their personality. Here are some of the potential reactions you might encounter.

1. Denial. Initially she won't allow herself to believe it's happening. She'll act in disbelief, astonished. You should give her a few minutes to absorb the issue.
2. Anger. Typically once the woman absorbs the enormity of your statement she could get very pissed. She's placed a lot of effort into the relationship and you you son of a bitch are throwing it away. This feeling is considered a normal reaction. This is a good time to make you apologies, fold your tent and steel quickly away. There's no need to "talk it out". This is your moment to leave. We suggest that you do it quickly before your caught. Use your cell phone to call a close friend of her to come and grieve with her. Later on her friend will organize the "boyfriend wake" and instead of a eulogy it will be specific and generic man bashing with liquor.
3. Bargaining. If your female doesn't have an anger phase, (or you stayed to long because you're a pussy), then you could get into the "bargaining" phase. Now you've done it, you're fucked. You're into the long breakup where you will now experience the "war and Peace version of why you need to breakup and how it's not her fault over and over and over. You have now taken the place of her good friend. This is emotional terrorism and like real terrorism, you don't bargain.
4. Depression. If you have failed our recommendations and have to interact with your female you can expect some depression. Again this is normal and not considered to be pathological for our reasons. Extended depression is a bad sign, but you have no guilt here. You dated in good faith and were professional and honorable through out the relationship. You owe her nothing. Beware of falling into the "Vortex of Victim", (see Chapter 2 Self Esteem).
5. Acceptance. The female has finally come to grips with the loss of her man. She is at peace and after a time will start to date again. The only problem is when people see their partner they tend to have some more grieving experiences. It is best if you can avoid places she goes for a while, (especially if you have a date).

THE RERUN

Never try to rekindle your romance with a woman you broke it off with. You made your decision so stick to it. Trying to do so will indicate that you clearly don't know what you want. If she does return you might think she's desperate and not treat her the same.

Conversely never go back with a female that's broken up with you. This is the same reason as above except you'll always wonder why she broke it off with you. It has the capacity to poison you relationship.

Reruns usually never work out secondary to too much baggage. Who did you see while we were broken up? You know you really broke my fucking heart etc. etc.

IN SUMMERY

As you move your relationships try to avoid the many pitfalls that are out there. Don't hesitate to rid yourself of the undesirable. There are too many others out there for you to succeed with. Always be the leader who sets the tempo of the relationship. Your guides should be honesty, Integrity, and above all honor. The person you're dating could be your wife, your partner and the mother of your children.

CHAPTER 8

INTIMACY

This chapter isn't about specific techniques, (there's thousands of books about that). It's about the sexual experience and its effect on your relationship with your potential spouse. Its goal is to help you establish and maintain your alpha-dog leadership. To keep you from fucking up the start of your sexual relationship with her.

A ROSE BY ANY OTHER NAME...maybe

There is one very important concept regarding intimacy. You are no longer able to refer to the sexual act as "fucking", "making the beast with two backs", "rocking and rolling", "doing the wild thing", "making it" or any other slang terms. From now on you should refer to sex with your potential mate as "making love" or being "intimate". Why the terminology change? Because now you're painting a picture of your future life with her and you want sex to be special. Now we know that this is all shit, but it's not shit to the woman. Remember where men think ... women feel.

One of the man's prime directives is to acquaint yourself with your female specifically to discern her particular tastes and goals. Simply put if we, (the man) can make the woman feel very good about her self she will typically reciprocate in kind. This leads us to the following postulate: POSTULATE #9 "WHEN WOMEN FEEL SPECIAL THEY WILL PERFORM SPECIAL". Conversely when women DON'T feel special they're not inclined to act special. Also note, you can bet there's always some future fuck stick in her office that would gladly make her feel "special", (while he's "making love" to her). Just because you've found a good woman don't think that she'll be immune to neglect and despotism. To keep what you got and get the best from her ...you're now "making love". You want a fuck? Then that's what you'll get, a woman with her legs spread checking the dirt on the ceiling. Who gives a shit what you call it so long as you're getting a lot of it. You pick. Note: Occasionally some women like to "fuck" once in a while, but this should only be their decision. They can call it fucking in certain cases, we should never use that word, (dirty talking during sex doesn't count). Additionally, the word "cunt" should never be uttered from our lips at anytime. This is the worst word a man could ever utter to a woman and will guarantee you a position in the priesthood.

CHANGES IN ATTITUDE

This is the one area that brings the most enjoyment and the most frustration for the male. Up to this point your relationships have been primarily focused in the pursuit of sexual release. You weren't concerned about tomorrow, or the girl, just the pure enjoyment that sex can bring a young man. When you think that the girl you're dating has the potential for your future mate you must now change tactics. No longer are you the "Road Runner" consistently seeking food from what ever source you can. You are no longer the "hunter" who hunted regardless of his appetite because he had to. You are now the "toolmaker". He's mastered his environment and hunts when he wants to and with a purpose.

It's important to cast aside the old ways of your youth. The new world man has a different agenda. Don't get me wrong. Sex is still fun and it's still a necessity. But somewhere in your young adulthood you'll want to single out a particular female for a long term commitment. Sex will take on a whole new meaning for you and your girl. How you treat it is proportionate to the level of enjoyment you'll get from it.

Actions on the objective. When considering sex, (which for the male is about every fucking minute), you must fight the deep battle and "prep" the battlefield. This simply means that you must place sex on a back burner for now. Let's put our "Captain Id's Pleasure Ranger decoder ring away for just a little while.

"PREPING" THE BATTLEFIELD

As we discussed earlier, when you consider a female to be a potential "Mrs." candidate you have to start her "training" almost immediately. That means in every aspect of your relationship you have to attain the alpha dog position, (sex is no different). With sex we have to use the power of no and "passive resistance". Passive resistance is the use of non-argument/ non-confrontational tactics to achieve a desired goal. As we discussed in earlier chapters the only control that men have over the pussy is the power of "NO". It's hard yes, (No pun intended) I know and it can drive you up a wall but when properly used can give you the decisive edge in the battle for control of the relationship. The sexual tempo is a "key" objective in this battle. You will be severely behind the power curve if you loose this. The following benefits will be gained by not running to sex too quickly they are:

1) The establishment of the "alpha" leader. As we discussed earlier, the establishment of the "alpha" leader needs to take place quickly and be maintained through all levels of the relationship and all areas. Remember you are the man and there by you will set the "tempo" of the first sexual encounter. The power of NO is your ally. Blow this and she will quickly discover your pussy addiction.
2) You're a special, sensitive and caring guy. Of course this is bullshit. We know you wanted to fuck her the moment you set eyes on her. By using the power of NO you've created this facade. It's to your benefit to do so and you must maintain it. You'll become different from the ocean of other men out there. It'll make her feel special and we all know what happens to women who feel special with their guys in bed, (REMEMBER POSTULATE #9, WHEN WOMEN FEEL SPECIAL, THEY PERFORM SPECIAL).
3) Sex is very special for you. By not stalking the "bearded clam" immediately you have allowed her to think that sex to you is special. To a young quality woman sex isn't "scratching an itch". It's a covenant hoping eventually to be sanctified by God and the institution of marriage. She's still willing to give it up to enhance and hasten the relationship, but it's not a free sample either. Sex to a young man is something special (sex to an old man is special). It's right at the top of our list! Later it will start to take on a special flavor. But this flavor won't be identifiable until later on. That's because right now the lust is so large at this point it "washes out" the new appreciation for sex other than physiological. Like

shinning a flash light into a spotlight. It will also establish the trust that you won't be fucking other women.

4) Too willing too early. By holding your sexual drive in neutral, you can examine the psyche of your potential mate. If she has a problem with waiting for your decision to have sex then she might not be the one for you. Immediate gratification, (especially in this area), is a destructive entity. If she pesters you for sex, or demands sex then you need to take a step back and look at her past relationships/behavior. Is she addicted to sex? Is she a "whore in nice girls clothing"? Does she have self esteem problems that she needs the immediate satisfaction of sex to function? Think about this. You're on a business trip or deployed for several weeks to a month. Can she function with all the added stresses of a wife, functionally single mother, and some sort of professional without regular sex? When women are 18-27 their sex drive is more psychological. They really need to be in love or some shit like that. Somewhere between 28-32 years of age they start to have a more physical drive for sex and love although still there, is lower and takes a back seat to the physical. In other words she'll want to "fuck" more than "make love". Now back to our question. If this potential Mrs. Candidate is pestering you now what about later? Will she in a moment of stress of whatever and cheat on you? Will she try to get you caught up in the vortex of great sex, (remember that the "vortex of great sex" is sometimes used to blur the true image of her)?
5) It will allow her to have a great memory of your first sexual encounter. Women place a lot of stock on initial memories. So you can use the first postulate "SHE WILL FORGIVE, BUT NEVER FORGET" to your benefit. By delaying the initial lovemaking episode, you will be her "Shining Knight on a White Horse". You will stand out from all the other men in her life. All the "demons" of great sex, excitement and special events will leave because of your proper planning. It will lay the groundwork for a truly special relationship. Oh yeah and lots of great sex too!

PENETRATION TIME

You have successfully "prepped" the objective and decided it's time to have sex. By this time she should be giving you slight hints at wanting to have sex. Passionate kissing, hugging, eating popsicles in a provocative way etc. will demonstrate that she's ready. You have played your hand,

(and probably yourself) well. It's time to make you final preparations for the "first sexual event", (FSE). Throughout your initial dating you should have been scouting out her favorite things, places and events. You've known her for a month or two, (yes a month or two). You pick a place that you think she'll like. Expensive isn't the rule here. It's the ambience of the setting. A country bed and breakfast, a beach house or a nice hotel for the weekend are some of our suggestions. Whatever you think she'll like, it's her weekend.

Once the place is set, you arrange the time with her. You take care of all of the details and planning. Then you "spirit her away" to your FSE. A romantic dinner at a nice quiet restaurant. Dancing if you can arrange it. Whatever HER preferences are. This is a "magical moment" for her. Romance is the theme here. Liquor is advisable but not too much. You don't want her to have a vision of her FSE with you falling down drunk trying to "fuck" her. You want her to have just enough sauce to loosen her and yourself up. It's a fantasy and you're the fantasy master.

The stage is set, the babe is placed. Now you fuck right. No asshole! Now without getting into specific techniques. If you don't know about the clitoris, the "G" spot and foreplay, then you're under educated in this area. You need to get a book like the "Joy of Sex" or something. Failure to understand these two areas and you're going to look like a fucking jerk. For additional help there is a website started by women for the benefit of educating men in pleasing women sexually, (www.clitical.com). This isn't porn its real education about what women like. Remember unmet demand is your enemy. Here are some general rules. You take it slow, deliberate and sensual. You kiss more than tongue. Light kissing initially will drive the passion for the woman higher. If you have to, beat off before you pick her up, (there's no shame here). You don't want to climax, (cum for you idiots) too quickly. Another postulate is "FOREPLAY, FORPLAY, AND MORE FORPLAY". That's pretty self-explanatory. There is a direct correlation to the amount of foreplay and the pleasure the woman derives from sex. She'll let YOU know when she wants "Pepe" parked in the garage.

Un-authorized orifices, (UAO). That would be the rectum, (asshole). NEVER, NEVER, NEVER are you to make use of any UAO here. This is an option that you would discuss with her later in the relationship. Use of a UAO would be a blunder of the greatest magnitude. Oral sex is at the discretion of the female. It might make her uncomfortable and ruin her fantasy weekend. This weekend is for her, not for you asshole, (don't worry you'll get an orgasm).

POST COITAL, (after the fucking) ACTIONS

Once you completed the sex act you are far from being done. You have traveled approximately 1/3 to ½ through the total sexual objective. The probability will exist that the sex will be mediocre. That's okay, first sex with a female usually is. You don't know what she wants, she doesn't know what you want and there's usually a lot of tension. It'll get better usually. NO worries. Now the thing you don't want to do is dismount. Let her decide when you are to dismount. Some women like to have the man stay right there, even to the point of sleeping, (or at least until she falls asleep). She'll let you know when it's time to rollover. If she does indicate it's time for you to dismount, then don't hit the fetal position. You're duty now is to HOLD her and CARESS her. Plan for all night or at least until she's good and asleep. Don't ever fall asleep on top of her, (very NOT SMART). IF you do then march right down to the local Catholic Church and sign on for the priesthood. Typically the woman will want to talk about stuff. So talk, talk, talk, talk and talk. This is fine so long as you don't talk about policy or make any decisions. Keep it light and talk about her and how great you felt with her, and wonderful she is, blah, blah, blah and other shit like that. This is a love moment here, so simply enjoy it.

THE NEXT MORNING

If you wake up first then it's your job to roll over and HOLD her. You don't have to do anything else, but the power of the hold is phenomenal. Even if you have to do the morning piss real bad hold it until you've HELD her for at least 10 minutes. When she's awake then you can kiss, decide on sex and then through out the day it's her day. No football, baseball or guy shit here. It's HER day. What you have given her is a fantasy that will be replayed many times in her head. It will get her through the tough times with you and tough times with herself, (and an attack from a fuck-stick). This is an important time and you have made decisive gains with your alpha-leadership. She'll be much more trusting of you by doing this and it'll be easer for her to accept you as the dominate leader in the couple.

GIRL TALK VS. BOY TALK

Once you've "made love" the natural desire will be to tell your buds about it. The general rule here is okay for general talk, never okay for specific "blow by blow" details. If your woman is shy about it then don't even talk about it generally. Tell your friends that you spent the weekend together and then dummy up. If this is the one for you then it's your job to protect her wishes and modesty, (especially if you want to continue to have good quality sex). If it got back to her through one of her friends that you were talking about it then she wouldn't feel special, (remember Postulate #9 "WHEN WOMEN FEEL SPECIAL THEY WILL PERFORM SPECIAL"). She'll tell her friends about her wonderful fantasy love making experience and will revel in her elevated status, (since most of them will have had sex in less than optimal surroundings).

SEX DAY BY DAY

AS you grow with this woman sex will become more common place. It is important to understand that the post coital actions are to be used generally for each sexual encounter you have with her. WOMEN LIKE TO BE HELD, TALKED TO AND CARESSED AFTER SEX. If it's late and your intent is to "rub one out" then don't. If you really need it then do the whole good sex process, (or go to the can and beat off). You only give good quality sex to her. Even with quick sex, she has to get hers and feel good about doing it.

One Way Sex. It's too easy to get into the "one way" sex zone. One way sex is the sex where you do it for the release and that's it. Have at least some intimacy there. If you do this it tends to leave a bad taste in the woman's mouth, (no pun intended). There are times where you both will want to "scratch an itch" and have a "quickie". This is different and fun depending on the circumstances. But avoid the "one way sex" unless she notices your discomfort and offers it up.

ORAL SEX

Oral sex has been on the rise, (again no pun intended here) since the early 1980's. Women don't "shy away from it as they did in the seventies. In the 1960's it was a rare occurrence. When you're with your "chosen one" don't pressure her for oral sex. If you really desire it then you should, early on, discuss it with her. If it's an issue for you, (like you really have to fucking get it), then this needs to be discussed early on in the relationship. If she's unwilling then you have to decide what's important. If your feelings for her is greater than your desire for a blow job and you stay with her then you must live with it. You may not bug the shit out of her for it.

CUNNINGLINGUS, (EATING PUSSY FOR THE UNREAD)

Weather or not she likes the tube steak you should become adept at "breakfast at the "Y". Women usually love this action, (again discuss before dining). Sometimes they don't allow it for fear of having to return the favor, or they have trust issues with their mate. It's not typically a thing done during the first sexual encounter. It is allowable if she asks for it, but if she doesn't then leave it until later lovemaking. If you don't know much about it then find a good book to read up on it, (again check out www.clitical.com). If you have a lesbian friend then ask her for some tips. Nobody knows how to eat pussy like a lesbian. Bon Appetite!

OTBT, (OFF THE BEATEN TRAIL)

As you spend time with a woman, (any woman) sex will tend to get "old", (never tell this to a woman unless you're shit stupid). When sex gets old it's a normal reaction in the lifespan of the couple. That's where the love should start to replace the lust in the relationship. Some couples miss this avenue and in order to keep their sexual life alive they try new and different things. This can be a fun thing if kept in a safe operating range. However sexual departures from the norm, like pornography, has a "dark side" and it can easily and quickly get out of control. Some OTBT items are:

1) Bondage. Lightly tying up your partner. Emphasis on lightly. This requires considerable trust but does have a considerable high to it. Beware of the dark side.
2) Roll playing. She dresses up as "Wonder Woman" and lassos you with her golden lariat. This may sound like stupid shit but it can be fun with the right girl. Beware of the dark side.
3) Video taping. Its fun but this should be a use and discard format like the porn. God knows what you would say to your little girl if she found a video of mommy and daddy riding the horsy. It beats the shit out of Barney doesn't it?
4) Swinging. This is a very dark side avenue. This involves swapping of partners. Remember the Van Damn child? This OTBT has no limits and almost always ends up in disaster. This is the dark side, if you like this shit then get help perv!

War Story. I had met this contractor in Kuwait who had a wondering dick. His wife wanted to keep the marriage going so she consented to get into swinging. He thought it was cool initially until he saw some guy with this huge dick bang the shit out of his wife in front of him, (and apparently she loved it). That fucked up his Chi so then it was a different story. He decided that he didn't want to swing anymore.

5) S&M. Saddo-massistict. Sexual pleasure derived from inflicting pain or having pain inflicted upon you. This is definitely a "dark side" of the OTBT and should be avoided at any costs. Once down this path is can ruin your traditional sexual enjoyment forever.

Flirt'in with disaster. OTBT should be handled with great care. We all have a dark side of our personality. Sometimes we have to protect ourselves from ourselves. OTBT has a high probability to lead the man or woman into the "Dark Side". It can give markedly higher sexual pleasures but that pleasure will come with a tremendous cost. Traditional sex will be ruined if too much time is spent here. We don't recommend this path for our readers.

COURTING LUST

All pussy dies off eventually. It doesn't matter if you're fucking Diane Lane or Britney Spears. You'll start to get tired of banging the same old pussy day in and day out. If you're ready for a long-term commitment and have chosen the right female then the lust will be replaced with the developing love for the woman, (see chapter 11 Married Life B.C.). Sex will eventually become an expression of love rather than a simple physical release. This is a normal developmental milestone and the key to maintaining your relationship for the duration. If you constantly court lust, (by doing multiple partners, excessive OTBT or cheating) then you'll give no room for love to develop. This will eventually break down your relationship, split you up and plague all of your future relationships. You'll constantly move from one female to another in search of the "right woman", when you simply haven't been the "right man".If you have problems doing this then you have issues and we advise you to seek professional help for your own happiness.

BIRTHCONTROL

This is where many males have trouble. As we said earlier once in a committed relationship it is best to wait three years before attempting to have any children. That's to determine the true personality/actions of your female. Now there are, God forbid some females out there that will purposefully allow themselves to become pregnant in order to hasten or influence the marriage to the guy they're dating. To enable you to achieve that goal of waiting for children, good quality birth control is an absolute necessity. Since you'll pay half of the cost of a child and an un-timed child can throw off your time line, you should have a say into the birth control issue. DONOT allow the woman to operate this issue in a vacuum. Unless you're shit stupid, then it's okay. If you're not then you and your girl should do good research <u>together</u> on the methods prior to selection. If she's already on birth control then sit down and discuss it in detail. If you're not satisfied this is sufficient now's the time to discuss it. Not when she's missed her first period. Some of the birth-control methods are listed:

Hormone type birth control, (BC). These are methods of BC that fool the woman's body into thinking it's pregnant. When a woman is pregnant her body gives off a hormone telling it not to send an egg down the chute to be fertilized. Some of these are:

1) Depo-Provera. This is an injection given to the woman every three months. That's it, playtime. Many women report they don't even have periods when she's on this. No red flag day. No I can't fuck you because of my period. Just have fun all of the time. The down side is that some women gain weight. Additionally, when they go off of the shots they sometimes will bleed requiring them to have a gynecological outpatient procedure called a D&C. Don't worry guys my girlfriend has had one and I didn't feel a thing.
2) The Norplant. This is an implant injected into arm of the woman every three months. It works similar to the Depo-Provera shot but it's an implant. Benefits are the same. You can't forget to take it, but you still have some periods with it. Down sides reported is that it has no break from the hormone. This can cause a slight small steady bleed from the Norplant. That kind of sucks for oral sex. Oh well, you can't make an omelet without breaking a few eggs.
3) The "Pill". This has been around since the mid sixties. It's what started the sexual revolution bringing out the poor oppressed woman out of the sweatshop we call home and motherhood. It is a hormone pill taken 21 out of thirty days. It does basically the same as the above methods. However it has to be taken roughly the same time each day. It has to be taken consistently, (for some women it should be taken at roughly the same time to be effective as well). Skipping a day, not smart, forgetting two to three days is really fucking stupid. Lying to your boyfriend/husband, while not taking them so you can get pregnant is a travesty. Since you have to trust her to take it every day it's an obvious downside to this method. The woman should also see her doctor on a regular basis since her body chemistry could change and the pill might not

work as well then. When taken properly it has our highest marks for birth control vs.: woman's safety vs. pleasure.

Other types of birth control. This falls into barrier-killer, avoidance types. They are:

1) The condom. This is a tried and true form of contraceptive. It has high marks for preventing pregnancy, but does suck in pleasure and ambience department. It does deaden the sensation slightly and you have to stop to put it on. When you're done, you have immediately stop and take it off before your dick shrinks and it falls in side her. If you've ever lost one, had to dig it out and sweat till she has her period then you haven't lived. However, with proper use it does prevent pregnancy and the post sex drippy pussy that makes the wet spot really wet.
2) The diaphragm. This is a barrier type contraceptive. The women in preparation to have sex will take out this mini-trampoline like device, fill it with spermicidal jelly, wipe the jelly around the rim and insert it into her vagina, (pussy for you non-medical types). Once in she will place it over the Os Cervix, (the hole at the top of the pussy). After sex she has to keep the diaphragm in the vagina until morning. After that you can start again. It works, but if you have a long dick you'll feel the trampoline that can freak you out initially.
3) Vaginal suppositories. This is a little waxy bullet that contains a powerful spermicide. It's placed into the vagina, up towards the Os cervix. You then go back to foreplay and try to wait 10 minutes until the thing dissolves. Then you can have penetration. Supposedly it should make a wall of spermicide to cover the hole and protect you from the sperm traveling up the cervix and fertilizing the egg. It has a reasonable success rate. But it destroys the momentum and makes oral sex taste really nasty, (like it tasted that good to begin with). It also makes the pussy kind of gooey too. If she's a little dry this will help though.
4) Rhythm method. This is a shit stupid method that someone created so the Catholic Church can make more Catholics. It tries to circumvent the rule that the good catholic shouldn't prevent contraception. Regular contraceptives are considered a sin in their eyes. Even though with this method you're trying to prevent conception anyway. But that's another story. Rhythm plays on the cycle of the woman's body. When is it fertile and when isn't it? That's the questions that launched at least a couple a million baby Catholics. Most of the Catholics I talk to think this is a shit

stupid technique that's about over. But there are a few pockets of resistance that still might want this, (like high school kids in the back seat of a car without a rubber counting up the days since her last period). If you do use this method then we advise your to buy a baby name book. You'll be needing it for quite awhile.

5) Coitus Interruptus. Commonly known as "pulling out". You wait until the last moment before orgasm and "pull out" shooting the "giz" on her belly, the sheets, her face whatever. It sucks because you miss out on that great last moment of pleasure you get from the blast. How romantic. Its only benefit is from making you feel like you did something to prevent this pregnancy. It has pretty much the same chance as regular unprotected sex. If you're tying to prevent pregnancy then don't use this method.

After you have your children then you must think of a permanent contraceptive method. They are:

1) The vasectomy. This is an outpatient procedure where the vas deferens, (the tube that carries the sperm to the urethra/piss hole) has a section cut out and the ends burned. You have two of them one for each testis, (ball/nut). It is really painless, (I had it done) and the only discomfort is afterward you have two cuts approximately ½ of an inch long to heal. You come home place an ice bag on your nuts and read for the afternoon. You take it easy for a couple of days and that's it. You're done. You have to "toss off" a couple of times in a cup and have the Doc check for survivors. Once he says the boats are empty of stray sailors then it's time for the best uninhibited sex you ever had. Total freedom from procreation. You can be devious and not tell her. It is a way to keep her honest. If she shows up pregnant you'd have quite a case in court.
2) Tubal ligation. This is a female surgical procedure that cuts a section out of the fallopian tubes, (the chute that delivers the egg to the womb) and burns the ends. It requires a device called a laparoscope's. They stick these tubes in her belly, fill it with air and poke around with little remote arms and claws and cut and burn the fallopian tubes. It's more invasive and dangerous than the vasectomy. But it's permanent if done correctly.

HONEY I WANT ANOTHER BABY

When faced with increasing age and her children growing up some women will want another child. This procreation desire is a feeble attempt to hold on to her fast fading youth. They think, "I feel sorry for myself. I want another baby", Children at 37-40 aren't that fun unless you really, really want that. Because if your 40 when you're having children you actually 60 when they get out of the house. That's okay if you know this and agree to this. It sucks if she tells you there's been an accident.... honey. Women will think that by having another child they will renew the relationship with the husband, make a new bond and boldly go where you didn't want to go for the sake of their vanity/youth. They also do it to hold on to a man too. It has worked so many times in the past. Don't let the woman talk you into this unless you want this.

FANTASY ISLAND

If you follow our guidelines you can make her first sexual encounter a fantasy. Fantasies never die and can be replayed many times bringing sustenance to a woman in a weak moment, (such as some fuck stick making a move on your woman). If you don't think that happens to YOUR woman then you must still think there's a Santa Claus.

As with any subject intimacy has to be maintained to stay viable. Never allow the daily grind of your life to weaken or dampen your efforts for intimacy. Never bang your woman, but make love to her. Never "beat off" in your woman. If you do then you'll eventually pay the price for your complacency and neglect.

A couple needs intimacy like a plant needs water. Schedule it if you have to here. You're the man and the leader, (not to be confused with dictator). If you find yourself and your partner struggling for good intimacy then seek professional help early. It's always easier to piss on an ember then to put out a forest fire.

CHAPTER 9

THE COMMITMENT PROCESS

As we have said before, this book's goal is to make the male reader cognizant of the developing situation around his world with respect to the gentler sex. If you have followed this book you're probably at a major crossroad in your life. Advice we would like to give at this time is "IF" you are going to allow a woman into your home, heart and bank account then we advise you to do so "honorably".

Honorably means that you are honestly considering this woman to be a candidate for the coveted "Mrs." Title. Being a cad, (fuck stick for us working guys), will get you into a hell of a lot of trouble. Eventually you'll get caught in your own "shit soup" and "hook up" with some woman who you, in a fit of passion, will marry or you'll get her knocked up and either begrudgingly marry her or pay child support. That's why we always advocate for you to do the "right thing".

If you're just out for a steady "fuck buddy" then it's your duty to make her completely understanding of that fact. It has to be crystal clear to her, and you. Never let this type of women "move in". You only allow a woman to move in if you're ready to consider committing to a potential long-term relationship with her. That doesn't mean that you can't change your mind if she doesn't live up to your expectations. It just means that you're "honorable".

THE DECISION

One of the main issues existing for commitment is summed up into three questions; “Can I live with her faults”? “Can I live with her faults if they get worse”? You have studied the female selection process in chapter 6. You have been made aware of the many things that can plague a woman’s psyche listed in chapter 3. Now we want you to look at her faults in an aggregate form and ask yourself the question, “Can I live with these faults if they get bigger”. Expect at least a 20% increase in severity and quantity of her faults over 20-30 years. Faults are like bonds; they usually get larger with the passage of time. It will be the same way with you. You have faults that will get bigger as time passes on by. So look at your woman, examine your observations and make your decision. This leads us to postulate # 7, “FEMALE FLAWS TYPICALLY GET WORSE WITH TIME”. Again remember this is a normal developmental fact. The key here is good selection initially. Remember: Tiny faults initially end up with relatively small faults in 20 years. Conversely big faults initially end up in overwhelming faults in 20 years.

Example: You’re dating a woman in her early 20’s and she’s already having some depression. You swoop down and seeing this poor pitiful sexy woman who graciously welcomes you into her world, (and gives you tremendous sex in the process). Later in the marriage the depression is barely under control. She’s constantly overwhelmed with raising children, working when she can, housework and of course taking care of you and your needs. You find yourself in one drama after another. You can possibly end up taking care of the kids and her most of the time. When the kids are finally grown you think you can enjoy life and she goes into menopause. Do you see? When people are young, (20-30) and unattached without children it’s the least stressful time in our lives. As we get older is when the stress comes in. Marriage, work, and children can all work together in concert to add to the “stress pie”. If you’re dating a woman who’s barely making it without this then you’re really going to be in “shit soup” when you start piling up what life has to offer. It’s cruel but you should aim for a “zero defects” when it comes to certain areas in a woman.

Don’t be too hard on her though, even though her ass is going to be larger with time so will your gut and maybe your lack of hair too! Always keep it in perspective when you decide. When you look at her through a forty-year looking glass look at yourself first.

Proximity. Now that you have allowed your girl friend into your living space you are the road to a full commitment. Since you have been a diligent student of our book you have recognized the actions of your girlfriend and have made an open minded, and informed decision for colonization of your world. You should now continue to institute your Alpha leadership and openly determine the status of your relationship. Your "relationship", (yes that's right it's a relationship now) is going to take on a new meaning. Sex, initially, should improve markedly, for she has colored in the first space of her paint by number dream.

The next step isn't really a well-defined step. In chapter 2 we discussed the nature of a woman. Leads us to postulate # 4 "WOMEN TEND TO LET SOMETHING EVOLVE… RATHER THAN MAKE A DECISION". As men make decisions, women will allow a situation to evolve. True they do help the evolution by influencing events that decide, but all in all they are prone to let the situation develop on its own. As you and your "girl" spend more and more time with each other, she'll bring over more and more of her things (you may no longer refer to her things as "residue").

THE "WE OR US" ENTITY

Now that you have changed into a "we or us" weekends that were once in your control are now determined by a new concept. This is called the "we or us" entity. You are now a "we or us". Throughout your relationship with this woman, you have to refer to yourself as a "we or us". It's for your own survival that you master this concept if you're serious about the relationship. This leads us to Postulate #8 "ONCE COMMITTED YOU ARE NOW A "WE OR US". Failure to capture this concept and you'll inflict numerous instances of pain on yourself now and in the future. Allowing your partner to hear you state any action, plan or statement using the Old Testament verbiage "I" is a suicide run. You must now and forever live in the New Testament for it would be blasphemy in her eyes of the highest order. To you it will be caught in an endless nightmare of her acting hurt and mad. Even though no actual fight/argument takes place, you will not be allowed to have any fun until you can appease her, usually by admission of guilt and some act of contrition.

Alpha-Dog Leadership. Now that you "made your first installment on the "purchase of a cow", you might as well capitalize on the event. You've given your tacit permission for the female start to homesteading or "squatting" as they said in the old days. It's in your best interest to set the tempo of her plan. You, as the leader, decided to let her "move in". For successful female management you must embrace the concept of "us" and look towards the future with her and all her inadequacies, (see chapter 6 Finding the Mate).

THE MISSION STATEMENT

Eventually in the course of all relationships the insidious moves and coy plays give way to a direct verbalization of intentions. It is important that you are prepared for this very critical juncture. You have decided to accept her initial colonization of your dwelling and your life. Her next goal will be to maneuver you into talking about "the future" with her. Conversations of this sort usually start after sex when women need some post-coital talk, (see chapter 8 Intimacy). Talking with her in this location is bad. Usually you're tired after having an orgasm and want to hit the fetal position as quickly as possible. You are more prone to "give away the farm " than at any other time. Put off this discussion by switching to how much you love her and anything else you can think about to get her off that subject. Delay this discussion until you can get on neutral ground and your head isn't swimming with post-lust thoughts. At this time you must take the lead and schedule a "talk". Successful goal setting is dependent on proper planning. Remember the old saying: the 5 "Ps", proper planning eliminates piss poor performance.

"THE TALK"

The Talk. "The talk" is a major defining moment in your relationship. You must be organized as to your own life plan before attempting to incorporate her life plan into yours. As we said in appendix A, "The Man in the New World Order", almost all corporations have a mission statement and most counselors preach that all individuals should have one. We recommend you read "Seven Habits of Highly Effective People". This will give you the necessary information to develop your personal life plan/mission statement, your couple and eventually your family mission statement.

Prior to your initial goal setting talk you must have your personal mission statement in place, (see appendix A). It should be detailed and painstakingly clear the processes, goals and objectives in your life. It should be clearly outlined with specified and implied tasks. It will outline each step of your life to achieve your desired end state.

THE FEMALE MISSION STATEMENT

It must be understood that this moment is critical for successful female management. Your mission statement essentially defines whom you are, what you want and how you are going to get it. If her mission statement is not compatible with yours, now is the time to rethink your relationship with her. If she has no mission statement she may not understand or comprehend what you have told her. You must educate her to the mission statement concept. Initially she'll think this is fun, because you're talking about your future and she's included in that reality. It's imperative that you keep her on track with this.

The female mission statement has many other benefits as well. By tasking her to come up with her mission statement you have the ultimate "get out of jail free card". If she wants to discuss "our "future together, you simply ask her if she has her mission statement ready. If she doesn't then you can't talk. It's that simple. If she doesn't have her mission statement ready she might not even broach the subject. Or if she insists you talk about it, you can respond that she isn't serious about "your future" together because she hasn't taken the time to finish her mission statement. The possibilities are endless if you need them. If she buckles down and finishes the mission statement to your satisfaction then that will signal to you that she is very serious about the relationship and not somebody who's just along for the ride.

THE COMPARISON

With her mission statement completed, the talks can begin. Start first by reading each other's mission statement. Then you look for like items and major milestones. She will naturally, (as you will naturally) want to reroute your process to meet her objectives. This process, can take the form of a love game that will bring you closer give you the "us" mission statement. It can also end the relationship if you can't agree. If you leave this task undone it will come back to haunt you! It will not manifest itself formally until approximately the wedding day plus three years. But it will come back as sure as God made little green apples. She'll love it until it conflicts with what she wants to do. So document, document, and document. Mission statements are dynamic and therefore can be changed to accommodate changing situations, (i.e. the unexpected conception... oops! Industry changes, sickness etc.) There's no guarantee that when you display a piece of dinghy paper years later, it won't hold any water with her. But it will give you the moral high ground, which has no par value other then perceptions of extended family issues. Then again, systematic review of the mission statement with the female can keep her aligned with her commitment to the relationship and to you. It could also be an important tool in early re-negations that women are famous for.

TO MOVE IN OR NOT TO MOVE IN, (THAT IS THE QUESTION...)

If you haven't already asked the girl to move in she'll eventually start with slight overtures to move in. This can take the form of verbal visualizations and blossom into frank discussion and if not satisfied fester into direct confrontation. Since you have decided to take the first step into a partnership, you must now decide if you're ready for the next step in your relationship.

Alpha dog leadership. If you both have submitted your mission statements, have agreed on a couple mission statement and you have observed no severe "warning flags" then you should make the decision, set the tempo and tell her you'd like her to move in. Failure to make this move will force her to nag at you about moving in. She'll think you're not serious about her or you're stuck in your adolescence and you'll experience trouble obtaining or maintaining your alpha dog. Never let her "nag" you on major issues. If she meets your criteria then YOU be the one to make the decision to cohabitate. Never let the major issues fall into her sphere of influence. This is a training point! If you take the lead and keep the lead then your life is infinitely better. However with great power comes great responsibility. This means that you have to recognize her feelings and needs without her direction and attempt to fulfill them. You are the man, biblically ordained to be the leader, then lead! Don't wait for the woman to lead! So you'll be the one to say let's live together/marry, (whatever is your personal choice). Make it your idea, not hers. You lead... she follows. This should be the recurring theme through your relationship.

Note: If she has deep seated religious convictions to co-habitation then don't broach the subject. Getting turned down doesn't help alpha-dog leadership. Additionally don't pressure her into moving in if she doesn't want to. Remember that this is your "chosen one". You don't want her to resent you all of your life by forcing her to "live in sin" with you. Find out her preferences prior to asking the question.

MOVING DAY

When the woman "moves in" you're in for a major shock. You now have to decide on many new things. Interior design is inbred on women like a duck flies South for the winter. As you feel you have divine right to be the leader, she has the title of the "nest builder". It is important that you allow her autonomy, (that means she's the deciding partner) within this area regardless of your feelings. The woman must change enough of the living area to change it from "your" place to an "our" place. If you won't let her change it then she might not feel special. Remember postulate #9, "WHEN A WOMAN FEELS SPECIAL THEY WILL PERFORM SPECIAL". Also if she doesn't feel comfortable then you might have to move to a different place. This is a possibility you should be prepared for.

THE MANS "FORTRESS OF SOLITUDE"

If you have the space, then reserve some for your "fortress of solitude", (FOS). This concept may not be too important now, but will be later on in your life, so you have to get her used to the concept now. In time you'll need a space that you can call your own. It will be free from feminine accoutrements, (girl shit) and decorated with your fine eye for the "male spirit", (no pussy pictures). It must be understood that she is "off limits" to her design autonomy here. It is also off limits for her work projects. Eventually when you have children it will be especially off limits to them. Even cleaning the FOS is your responsibility.

THE "BED"

If you have had another woman living there for whatever reason, then your woman must remove the "spore" of the other woman, especially the bed. The bed is kind of the woman's "soul". It must have a virginal sense about it. Women have a sixth sense about a pre-fucked bed. It will haunt them and they will never be free of the other women's spirit until the bed is gone, (preferably burned up in some ritualistic fashion). Seriously, get rid of the used bed regardless of what she says because if will fuck up her "chi", (If you want good sex that is). Remember postulate #9, "WHEN A WOMAN FEELS SPECIAL THEY WILL PERFORM SPECIAL".

OTHER WOMEN

Once you decide that you are going to allow your girl to move in, you must exorcise the demons of your past. That means that you have to throw away all of the "other girl", (OG) shit you have kept over the years. This can include, but not limited to:

1) Pictures of other women. This is stupid if you insist to keep these.

2) Letters. Clean or dirty. Very incriminating, especially if their dirty. If she finds any letters she will read them and you'll come very close to being punished for cheating on her. Get rid of them.
3) Gifts. If there is even the slightest chance she can associate a particular gift to a girl then you have to get rid if it. This will drive a woman crazy. Every time they look at the article it can trigger another session of the "court of feminine feelings". Why spend time debating over some inanimate object. Get rid of it, (because it will probably suffer an "accident" anyway.
4) Gifts of endearment. Any piece of jewelry is subject to this. If it's personal and your girlfriend knows you enough that you wouldn't spend any money on it then get rid of it.

There is a reoccurring theme here. Anything that has been given to you, or made for you by a woman should be discarded. Men typically think of these items as a value, an object worth using and nothing else. Women view OG stuff as an intrusion, an attack from the past from an enemy they know nothing about. They start to think that you're holding on to a past love that didn't work out. That she is the "consolation prize" and other such stupid shit. Even if they tell you "it's all right", it isn't. Things like this will start out small and eventually fester into some beast that the man has no idea where it came from.

THE LIFE AND TIMES

In summery the man should be prepared for many changes in his environment. These are good changes and he can solidify his alpha leadership by not protesting the normal desires of a woman. Be careful on what you choose to argue about.

Once committed and living together your thoughts should be focused on the we or us concept. When making decisions the man should be asking himself "How will this effect her, our unit and our relationship".

CHAPTER 10

WATERING THE GARDEN OF LOVE

As you are traveling though your life with your newfound female you must remember to water the garden of love. Now this sounds like so much shit, and basically it is. Remember, where men think, women feel. However you are in the practice of good female management. So you must at least pay minimal lip service to her and her ever-changing feelings.

RITUALISM

Once you have "cut" a female of your choice out of an ocean of many impostures maintenance of a good attitude is essential. The best way to establish and maintain good attitude in women is through ritualism. People, like children, (especially women), gravitate towards rituals. When growing up children develop better with rituals because it gives them a sense of security. When growing up a relationship rituals develop a sense of security here as well. Women are big on security because they want to know that the man will be there for them when they're big, fat and pregnant. It's an inherent drive that the man be stable for she is already planning her offspring. She wants the best deal for her children's and her future. She does not want to saddle herself to a man who will run out on her when she has a house full of children. All normal people want stability in a mate. If you're with a woman who isn't concerned you should look very closely at her past and her personality. If this woman is smart she will be actively judging your actions as you are hers. Some considerations for developing rituals are:

1) The "I'm home ritual". Regardless if your woman works or not you need to develop this ritual. At the end of a day and you return home to your "castle", you need a ritual that will give you and your woman a "moment of pause". That is a small daily re-enforcement of why you two came together in the first place. It also serves to signal to her that she is in fact home and needs to get in touch with her feminine side. Example: You get home and she's there. You kiss her like a woman, (not like your fucking grandma), then set her down and for the next 15-20 minutes "HOLDING" her and listening to "HER" about her day. As we talked about in the New World order Woman, (chapter 5), most women work, leaving no "sister hood" to talk out their problems with. They are forced to interact with their husbands to fulfill this need. This is the time to do that. You don't even have to do anything, just nod your head appreciately and make stupid soothing noises. You might want to throw in an occasional "it'll be all right honey" at the appropriate time. This is also a time for the man to discern any changes in his woman's attitude, (such as an attack from some fuck stick at her workplace). If he approaches this correctly it can also pave the way for good sex. Very few of her friends will have a mate that will do this, (unless they buy our book). It will make her feel special. Remember postulate #9 "WHEN A WOMAN FEELS SPECIAL THEN THEY PERFORM SPECIAL". Doing this action takes time but will head off problems that could invariably take enormous amounts of time.
2) Kissing on leaving for work. This is a common mistake. Remembering postulate # 9, "WHEN WOMEN FEEL SPECIAL THEY PERFORM SPECIAL". As we mentioned above when you leave your woman don't kiss her like your fucking grandma. You kiss her with intention, lips and with promise. Kissing her grandma style will leave passion out of her life. The "court of feminine feelings" will be opened and the stamp book starting to fill up. This will add another ingredient to the "cake bake of neglect". When it's done she could be ripe for a "hostile takeover" from some fuck stick.
3) Call for a date on Wednesday. You're not fucking Conan the Barbarian. Always give her time to prepare for her time with you. If you don't know what you're doing on the weekend secondary to work, then tell her up front the possibility exists that you could

get "called in". Judge her reaction to this and if you're called to that as well.

4) Your word is your bond. If you tell her you'll do something then do it. Don't blow it off. When she sees that what you say is what you do she will begin to trust you more. Women who trust men let go more in all aspects of life … like in bed as an example.
5) Remembering special events. As we'll demonstrate later a NWO man should have all the special dates in his planner. If you really want to send this girl away forget your "first anniversary" of when you met or some shit like that. Birthdays are mui importante', (Spanish for real fucking important). Flowers are nice, but this can easily become an autonomic ritual, (see next).
6) Autonomic rituals. Like common-law marriages these are rituals that are established without any conscious thought, and past precedence prevails. Just because you didn't formally set this up doesn't mean it isn't a real ritual in her mind. If you do something more than twice for a female or as a couple it has the potential to be an autonomic ritual. She will expect you to do this action all the time. Failure to break the ritual will in her mind signal that something is wrong or you don't love her anymore. So beware of the autonomic ritual.

When you break the ritual it can have the same devastating effect that it would to a child. Except that the woman has much more control over you then the child has. Remember in Chapter 3 Self Esteem? When a woman starts to feel unworthy she will have poor performance in all aspects of her life. Yes, that will include the bed. If you have to break a ritual that is beyond your control then it is best to replace it with another. If you have to talk about it with the female and explain it to her. Note: have a good excuse prior to talking to her.

SPONTANEITY

Men by nature are not spontaneous. We're planners and reactors by nature. Once out of the love/lust zone we are at risk for attacks by the women regarding our love for them. Through they require stability they crave spontaneity. They view our lack of spontaneity as a loss of love for them. When if fact it's just that our mental switch board is filled with other items like making a living, sports and sex. Women seem to have an infinite ability to generate these special acts un-planned and sometimes un-wanted. We as men typically don't get our bloomers in a knot when they don't remember "our first date anniversary". But women remember shit like that and we of course say how wonderful it is and how great it is that she remembered. Anything to shut her up to so we can get to what it was that we HAD PLANNED. So to keep us out of the "shit soup" we have some ideas for that busy male.

Pre-planned Spontaneity. The first step of watering the garden of love is spontaneity. The best way I've found to accomplish this is the "Pre-planned Spontaneity" method. This comes with such things like sending flowers with no apparent reason bouquet. Take your business calendar and pick at random four dates in the year. Mark these and when you hit this date call the florist and send her flowers. She will enjoy your thoughtfulness and the reward will be usually manifested in the sack. Remember postulate #9 "WHEN A WOMAN FEELS SPECIAL SHE'LL PERFORM SPECIAL". Women must feel special to operate at peak performance in bed. Never forget this. If you make the mistake of not making her feel special not only will you be fucking an inflatable doll, but she'll be filling up the stamp book for that oh so special day every time she has sex with you.

Spontaneous events. Like any good planner you should plan all of your special events for the year out. Like the special weekend, the supper nights out and others. Anything that can be interpreted as "spontaneity" should be planned out. Of course you should never let her know this. Then it wouldn't be spontaneous.

Date night. Even though you're living together, sleeping together and fucking very regularly that it doesn't exclude you from the date night. Just as when you have children you have a family night, you must have a date night for her not for you asshole. Courting the female after cohabitation or marriage is essential to good female management. She will enjoy the attention that you will shower on her and will reciprocate in kind. Make this a ritual for rituals are known to breed stability. That is what you want, a stable, happy and predictable female, (see chapter on the female psyche). Unlike the unstable, unpredictable, depressed and unhappy women who tend to max out your credit cards, fuck other men and eventually divorce you leaving you with half your savings, retirement and 25% of your disposable income until your children get out of college. Get the picture????

Suppertime. With or with out children. Supper is a time of community with your family, (yes, even if it's only the two of you). It's not a time where you can "shoot up the evening news", catch up on the latest sport events or watch your favorite sitcom. THIS SHOULD NEVER CHANGE. This time should be dedicated to your family in order to communicate the day's events, discuss new plans, or give her some of the attention she will naturally crave. It's important to remember that as with children women need a regimented life style. That's very different from "telling them what to do". Telling them what to do is being a "control freak", (not good). Dedicating the suppertime to TV- less discussion with her is creating a tradition in your house. This is for you and your spouse to integrate and continue as a unit. It will naturally be expanded as your family is expanded. It will help to keep you in touch with your children as you grow up. Remember the five "Ps"; you should schedule supper when no good shows or sporting events are on.

After the supper. When done you should compliment your mate on the completition of another fine meal. Never compliment her on something quick or meaningless, (like "you made a fine meal honey, when you know she got it from a can or it was frozen). Compliments should be genuine and from the heart, (or stomach as in this case). This will make her feel proud and generate some desire to do it again. NEVER LET HER THINK MAKING SUPPER IS A DUTY. She knows it's a duty she learned that from her mother hopefully. To remind her of it will only make it a chore rather than a labor of love. We want them to be happy doing what God has mandated them to do. Wine occasionally is nice if the children are out of town to lead into a night of "making love", (we make love not SEX anymore unless it's her idea).

The suppertime surprise. Occasionally when she least expects it, show up before she has started supper and "take her away" for a nice romantic supper. Remember your five P's (again make sure no good games are on the tube prior to planning this) so you don't get caught in a moral dilemma. Spontaneity and romance are virtues, (or shit to that extent).

Sports. We have to talk about this. This will piss off a woman easier than just about anything. Jokingly they refer to themselves as "Sunday Widows". It's in a man's nature to love to either play or watch sports. Just as women love romance movies and chocolate, we love the agony of defeat, (the opposing team) and the thrill of the win, (our team). But we're not the single entity that we once were. We're a couple, with many different facets to our face blah, blah, blah blah.... The thing to remember is we have to consider her.

The pre-planned sports Sunday. Once again we take the "alpha dog" leadership position and set aside a Sunday or two for her. This will to her seem like a spontaneous thing to her. Tell her some bullshit that she looks like she had a "rough week" at work and you want to get her away for a while. Remember you can pick which of the two of days of the season to miss. Plan for spontaneity because that's what women like and take her to some girl-shit thing she loves. This will be a labor of love and you should count on a whole day of sheer boredom. Make it your idea and plan the whole day and pretend you really enjoyed it. One or two Sundays won't kill you, the sex will be great and you'll have much less trouble watching sports. She'll go to work and brag to the other females how you left the game without notice to whatever it was you did with her. She'll be proud of you and will reciprocate in kind.

Additional tips. There are some additional strategies to remember when dealing with women:

1) Never openly criticize. Referencing our first postulate, "SHE WILL FORGIVE BUT NEVER FORGET", criticizing the female is a negative tool. It degrades her self esteem, puts her on the defensive and forces her spend time and energy defending her wrong ass idea. Then you spend valuable time and energy to prove your point. Criticizing has never worked to establish meaningful cooperation. A woman will begrudgingly do what you require, but everything will be recorded for later use. The first question will be "what will I get from criticizing her today"? Will it effect a change in her behavior? Probably not. Will it cause decay in your relationship? Probably so. No reasonable action is so great as to warrant a stinging tongue lashing. Doing it might make you feel a whole hell of a lot better initially, but will you feel better later when you're "jerkin the gerkin" because she doesn't feel like sex? Or she lays there inspecting the dirt on the ceiling?
2) Say something flattering about your mate everyday. Make this a personal covert ritual. Think up one compliment, (compliment = something good) to tell your mate. Do this daily, the results are great! Tell her in the morning so it will start her day off on a good note. Don't say generic shit like "You're such a good person". That sucks and she'll catch on to its hollowness quickly. You have to think of a genuine compliment that will show her you're a kind, sensitive and feeling man and all that other shit. Always be specific like "nice out fit", earrings etc. When you think about it, while she's at work, there's always another man telling her she looks great, how good of a job she doing and generally spreading it on with a trough. Remember our greatest enemy is unmet demand.
3) Look at the world though "her eyes" and try to anticipate her feelings. This is almost impossible for women change their feelings at breakneck speeds. But the alpha-dog is always looking, anticipating.
4) Don't be a "Volunteer addict". In life people will notice that you're a man of accomplishment. Everybody has community

projects and will want to staff them with quality people. It's good for the community and I'm saying don't do some of it but don't go overboard either. You might think that you're winning points with your partner doing all these good deeds, but in reality she might not like you devoting all of your time away from the home, the children and her. Keep it in proportion, never let anymore than 10% of your free time be devoted to the community.

5) Identify her "needs". This is a difficult thing to do when SHE doesn't even now what she wants most of the time. I want you now... now I don't want you. This is an accurate statement if you look at it from a female's point of view. None the less you have to try to formulate some loose association of her particular wants. Even if you fail miserably she will know that you're trying and it will go along way. It's not the gold bracelet she hates that she loves. It's the fact that you took the time to shop and buy it. Points to remember:
    a. Know her sizes. This includes dress, blouse/bust, shoes and ring fingers. Have this written down in your planner with any other pertinent information. Note: stay away from buying really sexy dresses. We've noticed this pisses off women more than pleases. Unless you're sure then play it safe.
    b. Colors. Women have special colors. Colors they hate and colors they love. Know the difference for your "impulse gifts".
    c. Flowers. Like colors know her favorites and know some of the symbolic flowers.
    d. Know her eye color. This is a general knowledge item. If you don't know this already you're in deep shit. This should be learned by the second or third date and committed to memory.
    e. Significant dates. I really shouldn't have to say this but remember the dates. Major Dates: Birthday, wedding anniversary, children's birthdays etc. Minor Dates: Your first date, engagement, first time you mad love etc.

What we have listed is the "bare bones" of what you need to know about your particular mates likes and dislikes. If you have been with a woman for a year, even if you're not getting serious you should know this shit. This is basic stuff. Yes it will take a little time to compile this information. You can start slowly by extracting one item at a time from each conservation you have with her. It will give you the needed information and she will think what a sensitive guy you are. If you don't then you're an idiot well on your way to being a first class fuck stick. What ever happens to you… you deserve it.

GIFTS

What to get? What to get? This has been said by men regarding women for centuries. We want to address this because it gets the man in trouble… frequently. As a relationship progresses through time and events, it is natural that you will experience inflationary forces in the price of the gifts. Men in general tend to replace cash with time and thought. Some general considerations regarding gifts are:

1) New relationships start the giving low. When giving gifts to that special woman start low, (not cheap ass hole). Example. Never give an expensive bracelet for the first birthday/special event. If you do that now, next year what are you going to do? You have to give the same type of gift you did last year. If you are hard up for cash and you get her a gift that's less, she will automatically think you're feelings have lessened or you don't love her anymore, or a myriad of other bullshit ideas that women come up with. But not so for the 4th and 5th anniversaries. Regardless of her thoughts, you'll be in shit soup for a while. So if you start low with inexpensive THOUGHTFUL gifts then you'll be much better off. Also remember that women feel that as they spend more time with you should give better and more expensive gifts, (and rightly so). If you are celebrating your 25th wedding anniversary with her a big ass gift is appropriate. Remember if you upgrade a present for one year then you have to keep parity for the remaining years. The key to remember is PACE YOURSELF.
2) Current relationships. If you have been giving a certain level of gifts in a relationship for a while then you have to continue with that level. To escape the natural inflation that occurs with a relationship then replace cash with thoughtful considerate gifts. A gift that shows that you really researched and gave extraordinary thought to her gift. In the long run that's what women really truly want, your time and time spent thinking about them.
3) Thoughtful gifts. This is very difficult for a man to master. Women do this as an art form. The best bet is to talk to a sister or a female friend who has roughly the same taste as your girl.
4) Consumable gifts. A nice option for the expensive gift is the "get a way". Give her a moderately priced piece of jewelry for a

special event and a special weekend get-a-way. Get–a-ways are great because they have a finite cost. A weekend today won't be out of site next year. You also get to participate in the special weekend. Nice hotel, great food you get to eat and of course you get laid. It's a truly "win-win" situation.

5) Long duration gifts. Once you've established that this is the "one" then you can consider a "long duration gift"/ Long duration gifts are those gifts that allow you never to buy that item again. Example. You buy your woman a Rolex watch. Kind of expensive but you will never have to buy her a watch ever again. Additionally, She'll never feel the need to buy another watch again either. You will have won on two fronts.

CARDS

Women love cards. Guys could give a shit about them. But to keep the women happy men need to have a card buying mechanism in place. Using your spontaneity techniques learned earlier you can do the same thing with cards. Pick out a sappy card for her eight times a year at random, (set your alarm). She'll love it and you'll love the attention she gives you back. It's that simple to accomplish.

TRUST

This is the most sacred item in the relationship inventory. Trust is the foundation for forgiveness in any relationship. As long as you have trust you can repair almost anything.

Trust can be destroyed by two methods:

1) Erosion. Trust like a brick can be quietly "chipped" away by small events not noticeable by the man. A little broken promise here, caught flirting with a woman there and it eventually wears away to nothing over a course of years.
2) Major event. Getting caught with a wet dick or a major lie, (drugs, gambling, pussy whatever).

   Actions on the objective.

   - For dating purposes.
     - Notice small breaks in trust. If a woman will lie about a small thing then they'll lie about a big thing.
     - Tell her small confidential things and then observe what happens.

- Inform
    - Tell her what your standard is regarding trust.
    - Let her know what the consequence is for breaking trust.
- Consequences
    - Minor. Only once, never more than that.
    - Major. Dump the bitch

Never break trust. As the Alpha-leader you should always "take the heat" for your actions. You can't afford to have her lose her trust in you. A lot can happen in a relationship but it is still repairable if you have trust.

EQUIPMENT FOR THE NWO MAN

We have said earlier that the man works best if he can plan as much as he possibly can. To effectively do this it is best if he has a SYSTEM. This is a pattern of holding and processing daily information for retrieval and use later on. We have found that rather than inventing your own it's easier to use someone else's. Some of these are:

1) Franklin Planner. This was the first of the "Day Planners" and still the "gold standard". This is especially true since the combination of the "Franklin-Covey" line of planners. Other planners include "Day Timers" and other Franklin clones.
2) The Personal Data Assistant, (PDA). This was introduced by Palm Corporation and is a huge success. Since that time planners have developed into a league of their own. It has the benefits of the Day planners but with the compactness of a wallet. It has the capacity to hold thousands of addresses, years of dates, thousand of memos and some of them can interface with your e-mail. The main purpose here is to make all your information about your mate, important dates and misc. data easily available to you. Many of these have alarms in them that can be set minutes, days and hours prior to the event you need to remember. Just think you're busy at work and your PDA goes off telling you to go and get flowers for your mate today. Or you can be shopping and find a ring for your mate for Christmas. You pull out your PDA, go to the memo and have her "vital statistics" right at hand. No muss, no fuss.

KEEP THE WEEDS OUT

As with any successful operation, planning is everything, (remember the five "p"). Always keep in touch with her needs, wants and desires. If you don't then there's always some future fuck stick out there that will meet her needs, wants and desires, (at least for a short time while he's screwing your wife/girlfriend). Your true enemy is "unmet demand".

CHAPTER 11

THE ENGAGEMENT

THE ALPHA DOG ENGAGEMENT

You should be having a wonderful time with your woman. She is filling in the blocks of your ideal mate successfully. If your female has met the designs that you "have' to live with, developed "her" mission statement, and you have had no "warning flags" that need to be explored then it's time for the "engagement".

Alpha leadership involves making the decision and taking the necessary action. She has made her "gates" and she has proven to be a woman of worth. Please don't let her "badger" you into engagement, (she will try). If she does her part be the man, be the leader and you surprise her with the proposal.

THE PROPOSAL

Like the first time you made love, the engagement is no different. Remembering our five Ps, (proper planning eliminates piss poor performance), You will want to set the stage for a momentous occasion. This should be done in a memorable place so she can brag to her friends. Remember; This can be a self esteem building experience for her. A nice restaurant, a scenic place or someplace that's memorable to the both of you.

THE RING

The ring, the symbol of everlasting love and obedience in her mind. This is another conundrum. You will most likely be getting a diamond ring. MOST WOMEN WANT DIAMONDS FOR THEIR ENGAGEMENT RING. Very rarely will you see something different. So you must take the bite. How much do you spend on the ring? The diamond commercials say a man should spend an amount equal to two months salary on it. This is all bullshit! (except for the diamond industry and the Jewelry Stores) The following are some thoughts regarding your ring:

1) Don't let her pick it out? If you let your female pick out the ring you're in for a long, difficult and expensive experience. Not to mention you'd need a skirt you pussy! You're the man, you do the ring buying.
2) DIAMONDS ARE NOT A PRECIOUS STONE! Diamonds haven't been precious for quite some time. But the diamond industry has done an excellent job policing itself. They have limited the supply of diamonds to such a point as to create the artificially high prices they get for their rocks.
3) The first step is to find out what type of diamonds she likes. Does she like round cuts, marquee cuts, emerald, heart shaped or baguettes etc. This can all be done outside of the jewelry store through indirect conversation.
4) What the diamond sales person will do (after sizing you up price wise) is give you instruction in diamond stuff. Diamond stuff is the criteria used to rate diamonds. Color, clarity, size, and weight. It's also a way to jack up what you pay for a stone. Remember these fuckers usually charge two to three times what they pay for a stone. We strongly advise that you to go there alone and learn all that you can.
5) Never, never, never bring the woman with you. First more than one choice will take forever and you don't want her to become educated on the diamond stuff. Most young women don't know shit about diamonds. We want to keep it that way. Her only questions should be how big is it? Does it look pretty? Does it have good sparkle? Or what style is it? Ignorance is bliss here.
6) Now armed with your newfound information you can go to one of the best places to shop for jewelry. The pawnshop. Yes, that's right the pawnshop. First if you think that the ring you're buying from "Snob Hill" Jewelry store is something special your grievously mistaken. All jewelers get their shit from diamond wholesalers.

They get it from other wholesalers or trades with other jewelers. Some of the stones have sometime been traded in from divorced housewives, lovers and just women who want to trade-up to a bigger and better diamond. So if you're thinking you're getting a virginal stone fresh from a diamond mine in South Africa you might not be, (and probably aren't). If you go to the pawnshop you're looking at a savings of to 50% on the price from the store. Besides it's fun to shop the pawnshop. Where can you get a diamond engagement ring and look at tools all at the same time? Don't worry if the ring is worn. You can easily have the stone set in a new ring for a fraction of the cost.

7) Size of stone. Now here's where it gets sticky. Buying an extra clear, colorless stone is fine if you have money to piss away. If you're a working class guy like us then you don't. So look at the stone with the naked eye. Does it sparkle? Does it look big enough? It should be large enough to occupy a space on the finger about 1/3 – ¼ of the finger. Remember the woman will probably wear it everywhere to include doing manual labor. It's going to get dirty; sweat on, covered with dishwater and eventually baby shit. So keep this "high quality" shit in perspective. The only people who pay attention to those things is the jeweler and the insurance company.

Speaking of insurance. Don't tell her about the insurance but get the ring appraised by the jeweler who sold it to you and get insurance or have it listed on your homeowners/rental insurance. Sometimes it does happen that she'll loose the stone by hooking the setting on something or the entire ring. Listen to her cry and tell her it'll be all right. Collect the insurance and repeat the buying process and give it to her for a holiday or event.

8) If she sees your ring and wants to change it. Don't. Period. Act hurt, act flabbergasted, pissed and whatever else you have to do. Picking out the diamond is your job, not hers. You're doing the proposal here, not her. Never, never ever let her in the jewelry store with you.

IF she consistently bitches about picking out her own diamond then take her to Crater of Diamonds State Park in Murfreesboro, AK. This is a real "no-shit" diamond mine and she can dig in the mud and find a diamond that no one has ever set eyes on much less worn on a finger.

THE PARTY

It's pretty simple. This is the time for you to build up your mate's self-esteem. So when you propose give a party later to announce it. It doesn't have to be much. And make certain that you don't get falling down drunk at it either. This is for her, principally it's her night to shine. Have a good time, don't kiss her ass, but let her know that she's very special to you. The sex will be great and it will put her at ease so you can get to see the real woman behind the mask.

THE LENGTH OF THE ENGAGEMENT

Time is the key function here. The longer the better. So whatever you can get her to agree to is good. Too long though and women will start to nag you. Never allow them to nag. Remember you're the man, the leader. Approximately one year is an average time period. Set the engagement to accommodate both of your work schedules for the marriage and the honeymoon. Women typically will allow a longer time period if they have a firm date to begin with. It is finite and has a foreseeable end. So if you think you need a date at the time of the engagement then set it now and set it long. You can always shorten it later if you want to.

SHOW STOPPERS

Never get engaged if:

1) You have any unanswered questions. This is not a time for doubt. This is a time for absolute certainty.
2) If you see "bad behavior". If she's displayed some bad behavior like flirting, extreme anger or any of the other warning signs then hold off until you resolve these observations.
3) Just because it's time. If you don't feel the urge to get married, then don't get married. You should love her and want to spend the rest of your life with her. If that's not there then wait or break up.
4) If she wants to "hasten" the marriage. If she's really pushing then take a step back from the situation and ask yourself "Why"? Is she having trouble with her façade? This is a sign to look deeper and wait.

ALPHA DOG LEADERSHIP

If you feel that this is the woman for you then you set the tempo. Depending on your religious/cultural convictions, ask her to cohabitate or get married. Don't wait for her to do that. Somewhere around 1.5 years of serious dating you should be considering this. Don't fall for her situations of "I've been offered a job in another state Shit". This is emotional terrorism and you don't deal with terrorists.

FINAL LOOK

Engagement is the final step to full commitment for the female. It's a time of fun, lust, love and anticipation for you and your girl. It's also a good time to "look and see" your girl in a more relaxed state of mind. Always be watchful to see her true personality during this time. It's never too late to halt the train of matromoney, (there's that money root word again) if you see a severe warning sign.

CHAPTER 12

THE WEDDING

At this point you have selected your mate. Tested her for the values you place high on your list of priorities, and she has met your approval. Most importantly you not only like her for what she is, but you "love" her. It is time to start the actual wedding process.

"HER DAY"

One general rule; The wedding you're taking part in isn't for you. THE WEDDING IS FOR HER. Yes we know that you're going to be in the wedding, pay for some of the stuff in the wedding and eventually pay to keep her all the rest of your natural life. But the wedding is still for "her". SO get that fact through your head.

Most women dream, (starting as little girls) about their wedding day. When she met you she probably started dreaming about her wedding day with you. Now that might seem a little scary, but women do that type of shit. So now that her wedding day is drawing near she wants this day to fulfill her fantasies. She will typically have it all worked out in her head. It is your job to make sure that happens as closely as you can get it for her. Remembering postulate #1, "SHE WILL FORGIVE, BUT NEVER FORGET", fucking up her wedding day by insisting on some stupid guy shit will be etched in her mind forever. Today's transgressions will carry double and triple word scores if you fuck it up. So your focus is on her "ideal" wedding.

Why do we even give a shit? Because Fucko, there are four major events that stick out in the sea of womendom. They are:

1) "The first time we made love"
2) Our "Engagement"
3) "Our wedding"
4) "The birth of our first child"

There are other events, but these four are the "bigs". Why we have identified these major female milestones are because they can be replayed many times in the female's mind throughout her life. Typically these times are when the woman has convened a session of "the court of feminine feelings". Good memories from these major events are like $1,000.00 "chips" in a casino. They can go a long way for you. So it is in your best interest that you maximize these events for your benefit.

Additionally, keeping in mind postulate #9, "WHEN WOMEN FEEL SPECIAL THEY WILL PERFORM SPECIAL", when properly managed these events can yield some very good affection from your woman. Make this "her" day. You'll be with her, but it is your job to make this the most wonderful moment of your lives.

THE BUDGET

Now that you're all "high siding" on your love and eventual marriage you have to come down to earth and consider your budget. Once the woman gets on "auto pilot" for wedding details the focus is shifted to "What would be the best wedding possible". This statement didn't include the words budget, cash, dinero or Euro anywhere. You have to gently "set boundaries" with your fiancée' in order to keep the cost to a realistic level. Always remember to treat this very gently for it is "her day", and you don't want to be the "fuck stick" who was such a "cheap ass by pinching pennies all the fucking way". Believe me this is what she could think if you don't approach it right.

Now the up side to this is that you can positively spin this your way. You're going to have to spend a little cash, but it will be the beat "venture" capital you ever spent. It is a tradition that that the father of the bride is responsible for sponsoring the wedding, (that means paying for it). The father of the groom is responsible for the rehearsal dinner. Don't start the celebrating just yet. If your future father –in-law is filthy fucking rich then by all means let his "little girl" have whatever she wants. But typically we don't live in the fantasy world and have to slug it out with the rest of the "lesser equal pigs".

1) Talk to your soon to be father –in-law and figure out what type of budget he has in mind for his daughter's wedding. After which offer him some financial help. Don't pay for the whole wedding but give him some help. You will be raised up to God status in his eyes for the remainder of your life by doing this.
2) Now talk to your fiancée' and let her know what type of budget her father can spend. If she wants more then you offer to fund "her dream" to a certain extent. This will get her closer to her "dream wedding" and raise you up x number of brownie points in her eyes as well.
3) After telling her this now you can successfully get her to set a budget for her own wedding. For it is now her money, (which is a combination of yours and her monies) that will be spent. She should be much more discriminating in her choices from now on.

The following are the general areas that you can financially break down a wedding into:

1) Dress. This will be worn once for real. It will then be packed away and taken out for show or when your little girl wants to play "dress up". Always keep this in mind.
2) Reception. The most costly sub-event of the wedding.
3) Band. Do you? Don't you? Live or DJ?
4) Flowers. This can range from a couple simple bouquets to flowers for every fucking set in the church or auditorium. Which means moderate to outrageous cash for some flowers.
5) Photos. This should be pretty simple but it is often not.
6) Building. The wedding site is important and so is the reception site. Money can be spent on either.

The main issue is that you corral your woman to commit to a financial range for each of the areas listed. Failure to do so will be punishment by monetary fines and multiple arguments with your fiancée' and possible family members. It will also ruin the "magic" she has about the event. NOTE: When settling her into a range do so at 80% of your available funds. She will invariably have some special shit that she absolutely has to have and you can get great "brownie" points by giving in for her day, (with the proper motivation of course).

THE BACHLOR PARTY

For the Alpha leader there is nothing more stupid than the "bachelor party". This is a time where all of your friends can get you totally fucked up and watch you make a complete ass out of yourself. Now if that were all it would be okay. But wait ... there's more! Most bachelor parties have some sort of sexual theme. Things can get out of hand quickly and now a days you can take home a permanent souvenir, (aids, hepatitis or one of the lesser STDs) if your not careful. Hell of a thing to have to explain to your wife how you turned up positive for something like that. Especially if she does as well. (sucks to be you)

War Story. Brad's party had around 70 people, (many he didn't even know). The organizers had charged at the door $5.00 and given a ticket, (it was 1980) to cover liquor, dancer and hooker costs. Drinking and dirty movies started the night off, and then came the dancer. In between each set the dancer would draw a ticket for a blowjob from the hooker. During one of the breaks some guys had bought some pussy from the dancer with cocaine, (we found out later). When the dancer came back from break she was really hot, (playing with a dildo and other shit). By this time Brad was completely fucked up, (courtesy of Jose Cuevro). The crowd was screaming and wild and had a pack mentality. All of a sudden someone started shouting fuck him, fuck him and the dancer, (still cook' in from the coke) drug Brad out on the floor, stripped him, blew him and then fucked him for the crowd. Now this seems like a fantastic party (it really was) except that the dancer gave Brad a dose of the clap (gonorrhea for you technical types). He ended up giving it to his fiancée, who by the way wasn't his fiancée anymore for some strange reason. Brad? He doesn't remember the event, but fortunately someone had the foresight of photographing him fucking this bitch while the crowd cheered him on.

If you're hell bent on having a bachelor party then here's a few "safety tips".

1) Have a "sane" friend organize the party. Everybody has a crazy as a road lizard type of friend who'll do anything to top his last thing he did. He typically won't want to hurt you he'll just get out of control and you could end up being the bill payer. Do not have the crazy guy organize it.
2) Assign two trusted friends to be your guardian angels for the night. They don't drink, and you can trust them to make sure you don't do anything out of "your" boundaries. Typically the bride to be brother(s) is a good choice. They have a vested interested in keeping you safe.
3) Keep the number of people at the party small, (15-25 people). Large groups of people can develop "pack mentality" and trouble can start. Remember the rape of a woman at a bar in Boston, MA. It was pack mentality that precipitated the rape and subsequent multiple rapes of a woman.

4) Never have the "party" the night before the wedding. If possible have it two weeks prior to the wedding. That way if something does happen you have some "wiggle room" for a solution. Also you don't want to be "hammered and hung" over the night before your honeymoon. You expect her to be in tiptop shape, so should you!

These are some of the pitfalls you can avoid. Always remember that the "buddy system" is the best way to manage the party. In the New World Order since you're having a bachelor party, the female is having a "bachelor-ette" party as well. Now the average woman has an idea that all men do this and they want their share of the fun as well. Women behave differently than men do when in situations like this. Maybe it's because they don't visit strip clubs, but once aroused in a pack formation they act like animals. If you doubt this attend a club where they have male strippers and watch the females in action for your self.

War Story. Grant, (a fellow officer's brother) got married to a nice girl. After the wedding, she had gotten pregnant during the honeymoon. This was fine because they wanted to start a family immediately. So the blessed event arrives and in the delivery room both of the parents were surprised, (as well as the hospital staff) when the baby happened to be the wrong color. Apparently, (after DNA tests were conducted) the "bachelorette party" had some of the same ingredients as the bachelor party above. One of her "friends" decided to have a male stripper arrive at an opportune moment. He did, and while the bride to be was very drunk intercourse apparently took place, (nobody including the bride knows the exact details). But she had this dancer's baby. The couple tried but didn't stay together.

What's good for the goose is now good for the gander. This is why we don't advocate wild bachelor parties. It doesn't promote alpha leadership, and certainly has the potential to be disastrous. If you really want to fuck around then stay single. What's new on the scene is some couples are having their bachelor and bachelorette parties together. There's no word on how well this new concept is doing.

THE REHERSAL DINNER

The rehearsal dinner obviously follows the rehearsal, (duh). You'll probably have a couple of rehearsals prior to you wedding. Note: Don't fuck around during the rehearsals. She's wanting this shit to come off right. Joking and fucking around will communicate to her that you don't give a shit about the wedding and associatively her. So take it seriously and help her when you can.

At the dinner, don't get tanked in front of her family, (or yours). This is for the same reasons as above. You should be very supportive to her, (not doting). You are now showing off your potential mate to the world. Since she's a part of you her success is now your success. Be cordial, be professional and continue to reinforce your leadership.

THE SECOND TIME AROUND VIRGIN

Sometimes women get it in their bloomers not to have sex for a certain period just before the wedding. This typically happens to first timers and is no big thing. They like the separation to give the illusion that they're a virgin again or to make the honeymoon night "real special". Typically the cessation of sex for a short period will enhance the honeymoon. Now this makes no fucking sense to us at all. But just be prepared, be patient, and respect her desires if she wants to go this route.

THE WEDDING CEREMONEY

It's now show time. You are purchasing your cow. Payments will be made throughout your life. This is a time of romance, (at least let her think that). You should strive to do something special, (sappy) for her. Some ideas are:

1) Memorizing the wedding vows, (usually one paragraph). When you get up in front of the holy guy have it arranged to let you state your vows without him instructing you. It will impress the living shit out of your wife and give you the "emotional high ground". It will reinforce your alpha leadership as well, (you set the standards, not follow them).
2) Write her a letter. Write her a personal letter telling her how much you love her and need her and how fucking lucky you are to have her, (leave the fucking part out) and give it to her just minutes before the wedding. Keep it short so she can read it quickly and squirt a couple of tears out before the event. She will come to value that letter more than a big fucking diamond. When she's sad she'll read it and it will keep her yours, (hopefully).

THE PHOTO SESSION

Immediately after the wedding ceremony you and the wedding party will be needed for the wedding pictures. This documentation of your coupling is a necessary evil and generally a pain in the ass. The wedding photographer can be a real photographer who has to do this shit to eat or some gomer who will have you pose in all sorts of goofy fucking poses for the wedding "year book". Whatever the case is you're fucked until he or she is satisfied with the number and quality of poses. During this session you will still have to be the alpha leader and support her desires to have the documentation of your love for her blah, blah, blah.

THE RECEPTION

After the wedding and you do this tremendous stress dump, and take your photos then you'll have to endure the "wedding reception". This is the time for you to introduce your "wife" to your world and you to hers. It's not a time to get all fucked up and make an ass out of yourself. Remember this is one of the top four events in her emotional life.

THE CIRCUIT

What is expected is that you and your wife should now make your way around the room to ALL of your guests. If you don't stop and say hello to Aunt Bea then you're going to hear about it from you mother forever. Make the "circuit" and then you're done with it. Then you can have some fun WITH YOUR WIFE. Again you should be very supportive, (but not doting) and focused on her. You want to build her fantasy for this event not hold up the bar for your buddies. Remember this is her day. Also remember postulate #9 "WHEN WOMEN FEEL SPECIAL THEN THEY WILL PERFORM SPECIAL".

THE DINNER

Some weddings incorporate some sort of chow for the guests. So you have to sit and eat shitty stringy beef or almost dehydrated chicken that you could have bought an aged steak for. Nonetheless you eat it and make like you really enjoy it. After which the toasts will start and you might be expected to make a toast. This is another golden fucking opportunity for you to say something really romantic to your new wife in front of 100-200 people. So get some help if your stupid about such matters and memorize a toast that she can be proud of.

The remainder of the event should be spent doing whatever the planner has in store for you. It could be gift opening, (boring) or they could start the dance. If you don't know how to dance, try to learn a few steps so you don't look like a complete and utter asshole in front of the world.

THE HONEYMOON

Again this is part of the whole fantasy package for the woman. Selection and organization is an Alpha-dog responsibility. If her or your father is filthy rich then they can have input to the honeymoon. Selection should be followed like any other operation. Some hints are:

1) Market survey. When you decide that this particular female is the one you want to settle down with then you should start a honeymoon marketing survey almost immediately for a honeymoon. Alpha-dogs are proactive people. Your marketing survey should determine her wants and desires regarding her honeymoon. Tropical Island, snow, beaches or Europe should be decided early on in the process.
2) Research. Now that you have selected your honeymoon site, you should be gathering information about different packages. Contact a travel agent for help. They don't cost anything and you can get a plethora of facts.
3) Financing. Yes we all live in the real world and must pay the band when it is done. Make a matrix of the top four packages you have seen that she, (and you) would like. Then run the numbers vs. your total budget. The sooner you decide on this the better. Once selected compare the dates for the package. The money you could save vs. a particular time of year can influence your wedding date. Don't let her do this. You are the alpha dog and this is clearly the man's job.
4) Reservation. Once selected reserve the package. Don't pay for it all up front. Make a deposit and make sure you can get a refund if the worst-case scenario happens.

It's not quite as important as the wedding. Once you're there you can relax and start to fulfill your fantasies, wants and desires.

Some ground rules do exists:

1) Don't ever get caught looking at another man's wife while on your honeymoon. This is a sin of the highest order, (you could also get punched out). You have persevered this far to give her the

fantasy of a lifetime to blow it by looking at a woman you have absolutely no hopes of ever fucking. So force yourself to personal discipline.

2) On the honeymoon night don't get so fucked up on liquor that you ruin the mood of the event. This is typically some of the best sex you'll ever get. She's "filled with the spirit of love blah, blah, blah. First time marriages this is a primo event and the women will be soaking this up. She'll also be tuned into making your night special because she'll feed off of that as well. So pace yourself and you can get loaded later on in the honeymoon. That doesn't mean be a tea totaler, use some liquor to set the mood, but moderation is the key that night.
3) Never talk on any subjects that may be even remotely serious. Never get drawn into an argument. This is a lighthearted time of fun and magic. Keep the serious times for when you're at home. If a serious offense occurs on her part, i.e. flirting then you address it accordingly, but philosophical conundrums are for later.

By following these guidelines you should avoid the major pitfalls that ruin the wedding event for the woman. Making her feel special is your prime directive. If you follow our guidelines and you should be able to maximize your wedding experience. If you manage it properly your wife should be able to look back at your wedding and experience the love and magic she felt for you initially. Women need this reminiscent therapy to remain healthy emotionally.

CHAPTER 13

MARRIED LIFE B.C., (before children)

Regardless if you are married or cohabitating you are now “operating” within the marital mode. For all intent and purpose you should be living a committed monogamous relationship. You’re doing what your Mom and Dad did, (or should have done in some cases). You live with this woman, sleep with her, fuck her.... oops I meant to say make love with her, and generally do everything else with her. Don’t make the mistake of only going halfway with this. Give her the honor of the position she’s worked for. For if she goes the “distance” and you make the final payment on the cow, what you do now will lay the foundation for the life of the relationship. Remember postulate #1: “SHE WILL FORGIVE, BUT NEVER FORGET”. That can, if you manage it right, work for your benefit.

ARGUING

This is probably the most important aspect in dealing with the co-habitative women. When, where and how to argue. It is natural for two people to have disagreements. Even if you were identical twins there would still be occasional arguments. So you must be prepared to argue.

Rules of Engagement for Arguing. The first rule in successful argument management is “Is the end state of this argument worth the effort?” It’s like the electronic battle games people play in the arcades. You fight, hopefully you win and move to the next level. But during the fight you lose some of your precious “life force” in the effort. Eventually you run out of life force units and die. That's the way it is with partner arguing. Each argument takes some life force from the relationship and your alpha-dog leadership. Is the win worth the expenditure? Are you prepared to lose to gain? Please don't confuse this with giving in to her all the time. We're not wanting you to try on a skirt here. We just want you to be the "wise" alpha-dog leader here and war-game the argument out to its completion in your mind before committing to it.

A technique can be found in the words of one of our favorite movies. Robert Redford in Cuba playing a gambler in "Havana". He said, "Its better to loose early with a winning hand so you can win later with a loosing one". The simple reason for this is that the steaks will inevitably increase with time and you need to survive the early skirmishes in order to conserve your forces for the later battle that could possibly decide the outcome of the war.

Defining your win. In a relationship having your way isn't always necessarily a "win". You could win a skirmish, but loose a battle. Your win today about who's going to drive the new car to work could result in her thinking you don't care about her. Or you're a fucking control freak! So off she goes to work to boo hoo to her friends. One of these might be a guy, (future fuck-stick) who'll side with her not understanding why that asshole won't allow you to drive the new car. Why does he always take the best stuff? Doesn't he care about your safety? Why does he always put you down? I would never do that to the woman I love. Seeds planted, seeds grow, was this argument really worth it?

Openly getting your way in an argument is not a good win. For remember postulate #1: "SHE WILL FORGIVE, BUT NEVER FORGET". Today's win can be a stamp in her mental stamp book.

Loosing your temper. When arguing never loose your temper. Loss of temper = loss of leadership. You are the wise man and you are always in control.

ANGER

We have to have a short talk about the feminine use of anger. When women use anger it can commonly be used as a "control" mechanism. More appropriately their goal is to get you angry. Now this isn't an argument or an assault on your Alpha leadership. This is an attack against you. You have made her angry for whatever reason. She now wants you angry so you feel the pain that she does. So she'll push your buttons as we talked about above to piss you off. Once she has you "loose it" she'll catalog this episode for future use. And believe me they have become "masters" of the fine art of pushing men's buttons. The longer you're with a woman the more buttons she'll be able to find. So when your woman is attempting to "push your buttons", you must anticipate this and be prepared for the attack. Leave the battlefield momentarily, (take a piss) to calm down, (or take a shit if you need more time). Always get to a "safe place" to cool down. The key here is recognition of the attack and the maintenance of your temper. Also remember that the more you respond to this maneuver the more she'll be tempted to use it.

Active Argument. If you have weighed the argument end-state against the cost and it is time to argue then you should try the following steps.

1) Determine her "end state" of the argument. Does she have an end- state? Sometimes no end state exists. She might be angry about a totally different issue that doesn't even include you, (like a problem with her boss and since she can't argue with her boss she argues with you). Remember postulate # 3 WOMEN TEND TO SHARE THEIR UNHAPPINESS. She might just be angry about nothing and want to blow off some steam. It could be an episode of "crimes of the sex". It doesn't have to make sense to us. It doesn't even have to make sense to her.
2) Argue only one issue at a time. Keep an informal mental agenda of the goal of the argument. Keep her focused to the main issue and beware of the "tangent strike". The tangent strike is a maneuver used by the opposing force to throw off the argument because they're loosing. It can come in various forms such as old argument issues, your past admitted mistakes, (you fucked your best friends girlfriend) or cheap shots about that person's history, (she had two abortions before she met you). These can easily degrade the argument, (and your edge) into a mud slinging contest. Try to keep the argument on track, if you can't then retreat and regroup allowing her to "cool off". Once you both have cooled down you can test the water for calm discussion. If it starts to heat up too fast again then abandon the argument or seek a mediator, (counselor) if the issue is significant.
3) Whenever possible look for the win-win compromise. This is the best possible course of action. You get something, she gets something. No loss of self esteem on either side. If you see this opening take it and use it. It's by far the easiest and wisest solution. Always protect your alpha-dog leadership.
4) If an "impasse" develops then issue a "we agree that we don't agree decree". It's kind of a failed "win-win" answer. If the issue is significant or she won't let it alone then as above seek

professional counseling. There's no shame in doing this, (see section on counseling).

5) If you're on the down side of the argument don't sell your honor out to win. We all have the urge to win, but at what cost? Remember you're committed to this person. If she has proven her point be the leader and concede. Praise her ideas and how you have seen the light.
6) If you have proven your point and she concedes don't "gloat" your victory. Again remember you're committed to this person. Loosing an argument can cause loss of self esteem. And we all know what that'll do.
7) Always end the argument reassuring her that you love her. She might try and hurt you, but being the leader you have to be the one to lay down the "olive branch" to resume normal relations. You have to, their is no point in keeping an argument alive forever, (besides you want sex right?).
   The court of feminine feelings,(CFF). We talked about this earlier. Again anything you say and do is evidence for her to review. In arguments never show your anger. If you show her your "ugly face" then she'll catalog this episode and extract elements of it for later issues. Yes women are authorized in their own mind to take snippets of events, statements and arguments out of context and use them in the "court of feminine feelings". It may or may not be a conscious effort. They may block out everything you have said after they hear some phrase or statement, focusing on that. Then that small fragment of a fact, like the tabloid editor, can be expanded and a whole new reality is created. Remember postulate #10, "TO A WOMAN FACTS AREN"T IMPORTANT SO LONG AS IT SUPPORTS HER TRUTH".

Be graceful in defeat but not so graceful that she is not afforded the ability to revel in her latest victory. In some cases, depending on her basic disposition or what ultimately motivates her, she may launch some emotional cruise missiles designed to hurt you in order to get desired rise. Now your next move is critical! You must display a response but it must be one of true hurt, but not one of subservient credit. Being hurt as a man is graceful or even gentile but does not render you subservient. So here she might of won the battle, but you have laid the groundwork of a successful campaign.

Remember an earlier aspect of the female psyche established that they are not tooled to look in the distance (the trail scout scenario) therefore think campaign and let her revel in the "close battle of today".

PUBLIC DISPLAYS OF ANGER, (emotional terrorism)

The key elements of successful female management are early training and consistency. The younger the woman, the earlier you start and remain consistent throughout all couple events the more successful you will become. It's similar to training a dog or a small child. Positive reinforcement for good things and negative reinforcement for the bad things. Now it's obvious you can't "spank" or rub your partners nose in something when they aren't performing as you think they should, (that would make life a hell of a lot easier though). But you must remain consistent in your couple's policies. If need be to the point that you share the pain of her punishment yourself.

Example: She has "acted out" while you were with your friends, (and their dates) at a bar. Actions on the event:

1. Never "blow-up" in front of her. Loss of temper is a sign of weakness on your part. She'll also get the point that her action had success. Poker face is the key here.
2. Determine what motivated the offense. Act(s) of omission on your part? Did you forget a special date? Acts of commission. Did she catch you looking lustfully at another female in the bar, talking to a babe while ordering a drink? Were you ignoring her? Now if it <u>IS</u> your fault, you must prepare to reconcile later. Regardless of the causative event the more critical event was her "Blowing up" in front of a crowd. This ploy of hers was a button pusher, intended to make you "loose it" so your friends and their dates see you as a big prick, ruin the evening and let you feel the pain that she has. You will suffer loss of face, dignity and your buddies will talk about you when your not there, (and thump your nuts when they are with you). Especially if you have your fight in front of them, air your dirty laundry and end up running after her when she will eventually rush off crying or cursing. Either way you might as well buy a skirt to wear and a dirty book to beat off with. Sex is out for a while, (at least from her). They'll relive the great fucking fight you were in and laugh. Now this isn't that important of scene. But if not dealt with immediately think about her acting up while you're trying to impress your boss or an important client at an important dinner party. Staffers with problems like big mouthed, low rent wives/girlfriends have trouble making partner or getting promotions early, (or even on time). These are TERRORIST tactics on her part. It's better to deal with this sooner rather than later.

3. If the causative event was you then you must calmly remove her from the public area and talk. This is a decision point. She can come with you and talk or she can stay and continue to berate you in front of your friends. Your only course of action is to leave the stage. If she won't leave with you then you go alone. Staying will only encourage you to engage in her argument. You can't publicly argue if you're not there.
4. After containment you can calmly dissect the issue and the events afterward. If this is a first event then you settle her issue first. This shows that you care about her. Then you work into the major offense of arguing in public. You explain to her that you feel that she's a lady. That public exposure of couple's difference is not the way you're going to travel through life. Her acceptance of this action is good. If she tells you this is the way she is or hints that this is the reaction for your bad behavior and intends to continue it, then red alert, warning Will Robinson, shields up prepare for evasive action. It is time to beat a hasty retreat and decide if you're going to live this type of life. This is a mental warning sign. A woman who flips out when in public needs to be scrutinized heavily.

Inebriated. If she or you are drunk then take her home and you go to bed. Do not discuss the event while either of you are drunk. Do not allow sex to occur until your issue is settled. This is a blunder of the highest order. She knows she did wrong if you left your buddies. The lack of you wanting sex will let her know that she's in the deep end of the pool. She could attempt to buy her way out of it with some really good pussy. Once you have snapped your carrot, you will as a reflex cuddle her for a while. You'll have lost your male superiority and the momentum to resolve your issue. You have to take the pain and stand your ground. Besides if you and her resolve your issue then make-up pussy is much better than cover-up pussy. And you will have won your first battle over the forces of evil. Failure to successfully resolve this issue will invite a replay later in your relationship.

The Runaway Bride. One point we have to make. It is very important for the survival of the relationship and the argument. Once committed and cohabitating/married never get into an argument and leave the domicile. This is a large mistake and will haunt you thoughout your relationship. If you're not married and she leaves you domicile put your foot down immediately. This is a line in the sand ultimatum. Once the female gets it into her head that she can leave to "make a statement" and get any type of benefit from it she will use it over and over.

Successful relationships require that both mates stay together and work things out to an agreeable solution. When you leave or she leaves it only brings doubt of where the other one was, or it sets up the relationship for separation or divorce. Men once the woman leaves have a tendency to run into the arms of another woman for solace or crawl into a cave and hide until we figure out a working plan. Once you have broken the fidelity of the relationship it can never be recovered. You can still stay together, still be married but it will never be the same in especially in her eyes. Let's say your married and your wife gets mad and leaves you, (a developed response that you didn't squash). You separated for a few weeks and have sex with another woman. You get back together and all is well for the most part. Now you have a deep secret that you have to keep, sometimes it's dependant on your buddies and anyone else that was there when you did it. That can be stressful. Two she found out about it and came running back to negotiate. Your back together, everything is okay, but remember postulate # 1: "SHE WILL FORGIVE, BUT NEVER FORGET! Your act of infidelity was cataloged in her mind and will never ever leave. It will infect her head, your bed and maybe be used for an act of infidelity on her part years later when you hardly deserve it, (see the "Grudge Fuck").

War Story #1. Carl was married to Monica for approximately two years. They had a child too soon, (he didn't have our book) and afterwards started to have problems. Monica became pregnant again, arguments started to break out and she decided to go back home for a while to see her Mother. After three months Carl issued the ultimatum come home "or else". Monica selected the "or else" option filing for divorce. Carl not having sex for three months upon notice of the divorce went out and started dating and getting laid, (big fucking surprise right). For the next 10 months he dated several women. They eventually got back together at her request. When she got back home she eventually got wind of his comings and goings. She accused him of infidelity. He said it wasn't that, they were divorcing, filed papers going to court and arguing over child support. To men they definitely weren't married in any rulebooks, but women don't see it that way. To this day, (they're divorced now) she still hates him for "cheating" on her and thumps his nuts at every occasion. Remember postulate # 1 "SHE WILL FORGIVE, BUT SHE WILL NEVER FORGET" Even though she left him, she refused to come home to him, and was divorcing him. It was still his fault. Never let them runaway to mama in anger or a in fight. Draw the line in the sand when you're dating. The runaway should be a deal breaker.

War Story #2. Greg was in a troubled marriage. They eventually separated and he started dating this other girl for the summer. At the end of the summer Greg and his wife reconciled. He broke it off with the girl and that was that. Wrong! Greg had gotten this girl pregnant, (reads shit soup). He wouldn't tell his wife because in the interim of the reconciliation she got pregnant, (shit stew)! For some reason this girl didn't need the money just then. But this is a fucking time bomb! Someday she might just serve his ass with a court order for child support. Or even more tragic, his daughter just might show up on his doorstep wanting to know why Daddy wanted his other daughters and not her! By the way in some states child support can be cumulative. Meaning the mother or the daughter can sue the father for lost support over the years, (potentially $900/month for 18 years). Ouch!

THE UNWANTED FRIEND

When in the course of the relationship there typically comes a friend of hers that you really hate. It might be a person who drinks with her and fills her head with little doubts about you or your qualifications. A lot of times this is caused by jealously of her friend. Sometimes the friend has no life of their own and hangs out with you guys "all the time" vicariously living their life through yours. We call these people "Psychic Vampires" because they suck you dry of your happy emotions from an event.

You can never ever tell your woman that you hate this person. If you did then you would be dominating her life launching her on her way to the "victim world". You would be stealing her identity by telling her what friends she could and couldn't run with blah, blah, blah, blah I feel your pain.... You might have to do this if you can't eliminate the pesky friend any other way. But always hold the ultimatum for the last card to be played.

The first step is to put on your poker face and as we said earlier, never let her know how much you hate her friend. When you see her friend either out or at your crib always talk to her and put her at ease. Focus on her and always listen attentively even if you really want to choke the living shit out of the bitch. When she's with you guys always pay just a little bit more attention to her than you do your girl. If your girl doesn't like it tell her that you're just trying to make your company feel comfortable. The attention you pay to her is almost to the point but not quite of flirting with her. Keep it professional at all times. This will put a signal to your babe that she should limit the exposure to her jealous friend. Is this a game? Yes it is, but if you do the honorable thing and confess your feelings to her you'll be a son-of–a-bitch for controlling her as above. Catch-22. So you make the call

FAT

This is a subject that is the most confrontational subject in the females mind. Women are obsessive. As we detailed in chapter three Self Esteem, body image is a major fucking distracter to good self-esteem. Weight issues for women a can start as early as age five. They typically don't like the size and shape of their breasts and nipples, their nose, their hair, their hips and their butt. Even if the female has all of these items in a perfect state, she would still bitch about some body image thing. Like the scorpion, it's their nature.

When we talk about women's fat we have two categories of fat. They are:

1. "I think I'm fat", "Do I look fat?" or "I think I'm getting fat". There are many combinations, but the overriding theme is she thinks she's fat. But in reality she isn't fat. Women have a myriad of reasons for thinking this way. Women "jones" about being fat. It's our Barbie doll society we have created. We have turned multitudes of women into fanatics regarding weight. Who is responsible for this? Men? Men like thin women with big tits. Women sell clothes with thin women, (big tits too). Women all want to be thin, (and have big tits). We are all responsible for the thin thing, (and the big tit thing). The issue is why is the woman telling you she's fat? Your job is to stay as neutral as possible and not answer the question, (see the "Moratorium"). If you can't get out of giving an answer don't give the Men are from Mars Women are form Venus answer. This is one time you don't want to validate her fears or feelings. You lie; you vehemently deny she's fat. Feed her ego, because her ego is directly attached to the pleasure of your dick. Be supportive, placating and understanding like you really do give a shit.
2. Really most sincerely fat. This is much more difficult. Typically she won't declare her "fated-ness". She will start to experience a loss of self-esteem. Lying won't do any good here. She knows that she's in the deep end of the pool and can only dog paddle. It's your job as the man to recognize this weight change and get her on the wagon without shattering her self-esteem. I won't tell you this will be easy. It takes finesse and determination.

When dealing with really most sincerely fat women you have to find the cause. Some causes are but not limited to:

1) Self-esteem issues. Yes here we are again! This is a sad song you will have to deal with women all of your life. So you might

as well get good at it. When a woman suffers some self-esteem issue, it could come from anywhere. You're not paying enough attention to her. Her daddy didn't pay enough attention to her. Her Momma didn't pay enough attention to her. Or it could go deeper than that involving sexual depravity and even possibly rape. This thing could have been hidden deep and didn't surface until she was older. Whatever the reason, you have to find out before it goes to far, (weight wise that is).

2) When women get a case of the Mondays on Tuesday, Wednesday and so on they tend to compensate for their poor feelings in other ways(see life is a house, Chapter three). Some fuck other men; some buy a lot of things but many eat their way out of sadness. A couple of issues regarding eating exist. They say that when the stomach is full after eating a large meal that "endorphins" are released, (endorphins are the body's natural opiates which are many times stronger than heroin). They also say that when a person eats chocolate it causes the brain to secrete the same neurotransmitter as when a person is falling in love. Is it true? It's pretty publicized and women do eat a lot of chocolate.
3) Genetics. As we said in the choosing a mate section, look at her Mother. Is Mom fat? Pleasingly plump? She has a good chance of inheriting her fat genes, and her mother's eating habits as well as some of her self-esteem issues. So if Mom IS fat, it's not impossible for to have a fit wife, just harder. Also remember to look at the ankles, (thick ankles=thick body eventually).
4) Just plain lazy. Some women are just plain lazy. They figure they're married and just let it go baby. Enjoy, you only go around once in this world so grab all the gusto you can. If you don't mind a slobbering blubbering piece of ass then it's your choice. If not then you need to have a heart to heart with yourself and her. It's come to Jesus time.
5) Post Pregnancy. This is a very special situation that you must give the utmost care to. This poor woman has disfigured her body for you to have a son/daughter God damn it! (see how easy it is to get into the victim thing?) This weight can hang on post delivery of your child and haunt you for years. It can manifest itself into self-esteem issues, (remember that).

Course of action. Breast-feeding. Breast feeding of the infant, (for at least a year) is great. It takes approximately 1000 calories a day for milk to be produced. So suck, suck and suck your way to thinness ladies. You also have the windfall of having Dolly Pardon for a year. The down side is that some when some women, (when sexually stimulated) secrete a hormone to cause milk "let down" during sex. This can result in "Ivory showers". Caution though: When the woman goes off the breast feeding weight loss program start the "together" work out program and your diet.

6) Home alone. No not the movie. This is where the woman is home all day with nothing to do except take care of the baby, have a little snack, do house work, have a little snack, do the laundry, have a little snack, watch some soap operas while having a little snack… So she eats because it's there and eats because she looses track of her outside world. Again we get into the low self-esteem zone.

Now it is the man's duty to recognize the added weight, it's cause and the plan to reduce the poundage unbeknownst to the female. But if identified early, and you "nip it in the bud" you have a reasonable chance of reversal.

Approach to weight loss is everything Possible actions are:

1) Exercise with her. Use some shit about wanting to bond with her. She'll probably like it and it will increase her self-esteem. However you have to tailor your workouts to allow her "spin-up" time to the increased workload. Yes, it's time consuming, yes, it kind of sucks when you could be out talking to you buddies about hunting, sex, fishing, sex and killing things. But faced with the outcome of being married to Moby Dick or the svelte chick you dated and married, well you make the call.
2) Declare that you're "getting out of shape". Place the whole family on a diet. Tell her you have had a revelation regarding the poor nutrition of the household and you want to change it. Kind of lame, but she'll want to believe and could support you in this. Choose a diet and get the book for both of you to read together. The Atkins diet or "body for Life" are pretty good starters. Remember, "suffering is the bond…."
3) Direct Confrontation. The first thing you don't do is say" You know you're adding a few pounds". This is the kiss of death to her and her self-esteem, (yes here we are again). Never mention anything about her fat while she's naked. She won't want to be naked in front of you. That kind of makes it hard to have sex when clothes are in the way. Direct confrontation is the absolute last-ditch action. Once "fat" is said it's like a bullet. You can't take it back. Once it hits then of course postulate #1 will raise

it's ugly head, "SHE WILL FORGIVE, BUT SHE WILL NEVER EVER FORGET! So use this very dangerous "silver bullet" carefully. This should be used after all above actions have been tried at least twice.

Once you achieve positive results from these recommended actions or come up with some of your own. Remember, weight gain can also be a symptom of something else. You should not only correct the weight, but try to find and correct the cause. Typically women over eat for a reason. Find the cause and your job is infinitely easier to do. If they're happy, then they usually aren't overweight. SO make her happy if that's possible.

PORNOGRAPHY

Typically pornography is a national past time for American men. It also can create many problems for the relationship. You must treat porn with the care of liquor. With in reason, (moderation) it's not detrimental. Occasionally some men travel to the "dark side" and get carried away. This can, like any vice become expensive, and the need for more quantities and severity of porn can grow. That can be dangerous to your relationship. If your wife/girlfriend finds out several things could happen:

1) Self-esteem plunges. Women view porn not as an idle past time, but a perversion if carried past the occasional Playboy. They immediately start to think that something is missing from the relationship and their "Chi" starts to fuck up, (I'm not enough for him, I'm inadequate, my tits are too small, I'm too fat, on and on and on.... Since self-esteem is directly correlated to good quality and quantities of sex this will invariably start the self-esteem "spiral of despair". During sex she'll think, "Is he thinking about me or that fucking slut in the video?" "Why do I care? Poor, poor pitiful me. I think I'll have another donut." Remember postulate #1: SHE WILL FORGIVE, BUT SHE WILL NEVER FORGET!
2) Expensive. Quality porn, (there's a fucking dichotomy), is expensive. Most porn starts out with a book, but if it gets away from you then you could end up spending some money. Now the Internet can offer you the best in porn. Live peep shows, chat rooms and eventually meeting someone as perverse as you are you sick mother fucker. If you're in this far get some counseling. This is definitely not "normal".
3) Children. If you have young children they have the habit of digging everywhere they're not supposed to be. No place other than a locked safe can stop these inquisitive little creatures.

> Having them find the dirty book stash could be very embarrassing to dad. Having them find Dad's raunchy "fuck fest" videos could work on their "Chi". Remember, Dad's a hero to them. They will naturally want to emulate their Father. Is this what you want your children to mimic? For your daughter?

If you choose to look at pornography then it is best to have a use and discard policy. Don't keep a "smoking gun" around the house for others to find. Especially if your OTBT, (off the beaten trail) porn, and get knee deep into it.

CHURCH

Once you are in the couple zone you might want to consider church. Church has amazing properties that people don't realize. First it's of course spiritual, good for the soul and that never hurts. It's also good for the relationship and female. Going to church allows the woman significance in her life. It gives her friends, a support system and an avenue for her spare time. If she is the type to not work, then church is definitely the answer. This will get her out of the house and do good deeds for God, community and country. If she's busy, then she's not at home exploring your transgressions/faults. It also gives her a good idea of what a good wife should do and a reference of what a good wife should not do. God has developed a great plan for the world, (it's the best owners manual for couple happiness). It does not encourage women on their own with the help of the ex-husband paying money and giving her every other weekend off from the kids. Many churches also have good childcare facilities, knowing that the parents come to church, and they can develop the children as well. It's a win, win situation establishing yourselves in the church.

HOLIDAYS

Once you're together either as cohabitants or man and wife you will invariably develop the "holiday crisis". This is precipitated by the families of the couple. In all good nature you must have this thought out ahead of time. Holiday crisis will take any fun out of the holiday even if she gives you a Christmas blowjob. What happens is that now the two of you are effectively one you must be "shared". To do this effectively and avoid the hurt painful looks on either of your families you develop a "holiday plan". This will be similar to a divorce settlement of holiday visits. Set down your lovely mate and work this out prior to the invitations being sent. You as the male must set the tempo for this. Be fair and equitable with the assignments. If you're in the same town then always plan a "drive by" visit after your family's supper. This helps the woman adjust to the missed family event and score big points for you with her. A good plan and possible holiday drive bys and the "holiday crisis" will be just a vicious rumor.

BIRTHDAYS

This is a very important section. Women are sensitive to birthdays anyway. They would rather forget them, but by God you had better never. This is a time for you to shine. It's not the expense you incur; it's the premeditation you take for her "special day". This day can be an attack on her self-esteem or a recharge. It depends how you handle it. Some ideas are but aren't limited to:

1) Start the day off with breakfast in bed, (if time allows). If not then a card on the pillow. This will put her in a good mood. Homemade cards are a plus if they're good. Something scribbled on a napkin isn't good.
2) Flowers at work. Public acts of affection allow her to brag about how wonderful her husband is. It also allows her to feel that SHE is worth more as well. Remember SHE MUST FEEL GOOD ABOUT HER SELF. It also has the secondary effect to show any men in the workplace that someone is keeping tabs on her.
3) Dinner. If her birthday falls on a weekend then make it a sleep over. Girls will love a sleep over in a nice hotel. You must make all the arrangements to include packing her overnight bag. All she should have to do is being picked up at work and taken to her fantasy night. Don't hold back on this. Wine, dine and have sex.
4) Special weekends. Extend the above if possible to a whole weekend. Women desperately want your time rather than your money, (prior to divorce). Time is typically their currency. Even though this could set you back some now is the time to do such a thing.

Now we advise that you don't get into the jewelry thing too quickly. If you use the fantasy weekend it's far more fun, and more memorable than a piece of jewelry. Besides jewelry is a quantifiable thing. Each year you will almost be expected to increase the prize/size. It's a never-ending battle. Now the weekend is typically the same and you can participate as well. It's also a given that your supposed to have sex during the weekend. Note: on the fantasy weekend, don't sit and watch a sports game on TV.

If you're that into the game record it. Remember postulate #1: WOMEN FORGIVE BUT THEY WILL NEVER FORGET.

We know that this is a lot of shit, but it's one fucking day a year. Deal with it! Use this tactic on anniversary's the same way.

MAJOR PURCHASES

Major purchases can have two purposes. They in the eyes of the man serve a particular function. In the eyes of the woman major purchases can appear to have more than it's intended purpose. The man must be sensitive to these areas and maneuver through them to satisfy his rational needs and her more emotional needs.

The house purchase is the most important purchase that young couples engage in. To the man it's his castle and MUST be functional, practical and affordable. To her it's her NEST, capable of housing her yet to be conceived offspring. As we said earlier, the woman is typically in-charge of the nest and we must let her think that all through the buying process. Deny her this God given right and you will be sending a off a SCUD missile to her self esteem that will be very hard if not impossible to repair.

The car is another issue. This is typically "your lane". Now the wise man will incorporate her feelings and input about what type of vehicle is needed. You are the decision maker though. Do not relinquish this position. That doesn't mean that you go out and buy a Corvette for a family of four people just because you can. Not a smart action. But don't allow her to pick the brand, the style or the mechanical offerings of the vehicle. If you buy new then you can allow her to do the color and maybe the seating of the car. Now if you're smart you'll take the "old car" and use it for yourself. This shows that you care to give her the best for her protection. It will also leave you in a position to lay the ground work for the boat, motor home or motorcycle purchase in the future. If you become a true master of relationships she will be encouraging you to buy the Corvette.

War Story. Paul and Cindy have been married for twenty years and is still on their honeymoon. This was a conscious decision on their part. Both are masters of relationships. For example Paul was working lots of overtime. His wife was home with the kids but she knew that he was bustin his ass for the good of the family. Since they had all the overtime she took some money and when he finished the assignment gave him tickets to go big game hunting out west. How many wives would do that for their husbands? Conversely Paul one day realized that his wife was bustin her ass with the kids. So he secures luxury tickets and accommodations for her and her Mother to go on a fantasy shopping trip. He had all the kids babysitting time arranged and all she had to do was simply pack and go for three days, (plus he gave her $1,000 to spend).

MARRIED LIFE

Once you have made the final purchase on the cow you now own a brand new bride. The new bride doesn't come with an owners manual nor does it have purchasable upgrades to it's central processing unit. What you have is what you have. You can increase it's data base in some areas, but remember memory is non-erasable. In laymen's terms SHE WILL NEVER FORGET. We wish to talk about some pitfalls that become the man during his initial forays into his married life.

Once married your life with your female will be different. Your relationship with her is different, everything is now different. You are bound together spiritually, morally, ethically and most importantly financially. What you do now will have the potential to permanently affect you, (mentally and financially) for the rest of your life.

MARRIAGE + 3

Through out your dating years, (yes years plural is always a good thing) your female has been on a search for a "holy grail". This is the coveted state of "matrimoney". This is the wrong spelling but it emphasizes the root word here "-money". Now that she has achieved this status she can relax. She's made it, whew! Time for a break, huh? We recommend that this is the time to watch the closest. During this time of sex, bonding, sex, fun, sex .....you're learning about each other to a more intense level than ever before. What you have learned in this book should be put to use at this time.

Most people can put up a façade for a time, especially if they don't live with that person. Once in a committed relationship, (both emotionally and financially) the woman has the ability to relax her façade and you can see the "real" person eventually. We recommend that you wait at least three years before entertaining any thoughts of children. If you can wait longer then fine, but it is our official advise to wait at least the three years.

Why three years? Because most people can't keep up a false façade for that long. It will invariably sneak out and their true colors will be discovered. Major self esteem issues, personality disorders and mental instability can be discovered during this time.

What to do? So what if you find out that your loved one has some depressive type disorder that she just happened to forget about. She'll explain it away as "no big deal", but now your watching her take her "medicine" each and every day wondering what the fuck is she taking? As we said earlier, it is our goal to make the reader aware of the situation. What you do is your decision, not ours. But remember that your decision can affect not only you, your finances, your retirement and most importantly your children potentially for generations.

War Story. Ben was a fellow RN who met Kim (another RN) dated her and eventually marrying her. They were in their early thirties and wanted children as soon as possible. After their second child was born, (within two years of their marriage) she had casually informed him that her estranged mother didn't just runaway as she had said. She was actually committed permanently in a mental hospital as a "paranoid schizophrenic". Upon questioning she didn't feel that it was a big thing, just a "family embarrassment". He did his research and found out that mental illness, (especially schizophrenia is considered "familial", (meaning it can be potentially passed genetically to children). But this is a decision that he didn't get to make. His wife is okay for the most part, but now he's waiting to see if the gene will be expressed in his children, (schizophrenia usually is seen around young adult hood). If his kids are responsible then they shouldn't have children.

As with all of our advice "time is the penicillin for all cures". The first three yeas is crucial for the final "cut" of your female. This is defiantly not romantic, cold calculating and at best brutal. But so is having your children potential schizophrenics, bi-polar or depressed. If a woman is hiding "something" then you should have had access to that knowledge early. But since she didn't you can act however you feel once it is discovered. Once children are involved divorce is debilitatingly brutal and very, very expensive.

LUST VS. LOVE

After your third year the lustful passionate lovemaking should be changing. The animal lust you have experienced should start to be replaced with a developing deep love. She isn't just a sexual partner or girlfriend, she's your best friend and confidant. She should be developing into your closest relative to you. If you don't feel that happening then you need to problem solve on yourself first, then your mate. Don't have kids unless you're heading in a favorable direction.

TO BE OR NOT TO BE … a parent

The decision to have children is not an easy one. Your primary goal for children should be preparing them for survival in the outside world. You don't want them living at home until they're 45. That's not considered normal. If you're not prepared to see this task through to completion then hold off having children. Frank discussion with all the inclusions should take place. Some considerations are:

1) The "twenty year" rule. When planning to have children you should always add 20 years to your current age. That's how old you will be when you have this child raised. It's good for planning your retirement, college and all your future endeavors.
2) The "child support rule". Yes, this has to be considered. If "shit happens" what will be the cost and impact of the resultant child support to your overall life plan? A general rule of thumb is 20% of your net for the first child and 5% for each additional child. $55,000 - $65,000 year income will run you around $1,000 a month until the child turns 18 plus college tuition assistance and healthcare. Also add travel costs and child care until their older. You still have to pay child support when they're with you.
3) College Fund. Start now. College is as important to your child as high school was to a 1960 person. It's a bare minimum of education to insure your child's success. And it isn't cheap. If you start now the cost is less.
4) Total Cost of raising a child. According to "Smart Money", the US Department of Agriculture estimated that in 1995, a child cost approximately $145,320.00 in a middle-income family over 18 years. A more realistic estimate of expenses from birth to college, might be closer to $400,000.00, (this includes delivery, hospital stay, baby furniture, clothes, food, diapers, daycare, toys, books and well-baby visits and immunizations). Now what's the real costs? Try maybe around $200,000.00. What we are trying to say here is kids cost a lot. This is a large investment with a potential for great gain or a monumental fuck-up. Remember Steve Martin in the movie "Parent Hood"? As he sat in the office of the principle he was imagining his child graduating Suma Cum Laude from college telling his Dad how he helped him. Then he had a nightmare detailing his son as a sniper on the college church steeple. Both are real fears that need consideration. Basically if you decide to have a child, then fucking <u>be</u> there for that child.

Invest your time because in the long run that's what makes the person. Not a piece of paper with a picture of Ben Franklin on it.

THE NEVER ENDING GAME SHOW OF LIFE

Throughout the course of your commitment and possibly marriage, you will get asked many "hypothetical" and real questions. This is like the old time game shows on TV. They ask stupid fucking "feminine" questions and we have to answer them as best we can. To this day we have never understood why women ask these frivolous, meaningless questions. One possibility is that your answer will make them feel special. Remember Postulate # 9, "WHEN WOMEN FEEL SPECIAL THEY WILL ACT SPECIAL" failure to make a woman feel special will result in moody snits and poor quality sex. Your answers may also be recorded in the "feminine feelings" logbook of your relationship. Like anything else you say or do it can be held against you in a court of "feminine feelings".

THE MORITORIUM

Now there are some "feminine" questions that need to be avoided at all costs. Examples of this are "Do you like my hair?" Or "do I look fat?" or (if married) "will you re-marry if I die"? There is no correct answer to these types of questions. Our advice is simply never answer them. Now "dummying up" and saying nothing is as bad as answering her question. She will undoubtedly think you don't care about her enough to give her an answer. So we have some guidance to give her a measured pre-positioned response to acknowledge her and successfully avoid answering the question. If forced into an answer always be vague in any response.

Do you like my new hair? Now it is clear that the woman is asking the hair question to either validate her new hair or the fat question to counter her fat paranoia, (which all women have), her fears of getting older or just get a compliment, (to feel special). If you tell her you love her new hair then she might wonder what you didn't like about her old hair. If she changed the color of her hair and you stupidly tell her you like it, then she might think, (but not necessarily ask, "What old girlfriend am I reminding him of"?

For the hair question, the answer is, "your hair doesn't matter to me, its not what attracts me to you, you could be missing hair and it wouldn't matter". Never deviate from this answer!

Having dodged the hair question you must be prepared for the follow-on "bonus" question. You must have a follow-on answer to the potential next question. "What is it about me that you are so attracted to?" You immediately say without hesitation your EYES!!! You can even pontificate on this with such bullshit as "the eyes are the route to a person's soul, (or other such similar shit). This answer offers her no wiggle room (note: remember to know her eye color!!!!!!). Do your research here and have a memorized scripted answer.

"Do I look fat?" This is another minefield that must be handled very carefully. Remember her self esteem and the direct correlation of her self esteem to your dick. If you tell her she's thin and she doesn't feel she's thin then you're a liar. If you validate that she's fat you have scored a direct hit on her self-esteem and you will indirectly pay for her loss of self-esteem later.

The best answer for this questions is simple. "Who's filled your head with this nonsense?" or "Girth is a function of numbers and I don't measure you that way…love is immeasurable" or some other meaningless feminine drivel. It is dangerous to give off any answer that might be considered as "affirmative".

If I die will you ever get remarried? Why women ask this shit is beyond us! If you say what you think she might want to hear, you could say something like "You're the only woman I would ever marry". That would get the bonus question of "Why? Don't you like marriage?" You have tried to say something that you think would be sweet only to find that you have now bashed the whole institution of marriage! This is why answering feminine questions is like "Catch-22"

The answer to the re-marriage question is, "I'm not going to have this conversation with you it is morbid and depressing". You must act noticeably distressed about death and she'll leave this area alone. If forced to answer use any response that allows you to NEVER ANSWER THEM. You have enough to do in life without taking time out to answer and possibly argue about these feminine philosophical questions.

OVERALL

Marriage BC can be a time of magic, fun and tremendous feelings for your woman. You're enjoying the folly of love and lust that will eventually usher in the deep emotional love that will bridge you to a long established relationship. Never give up leadership for sex, (even if it hurts). Always act with honor in the relationship and always wait for at least three years for having a child. If you see warning signs take a step back, look hard and if necessary leave. Hard as it may be it's better to cut your losses without the emotional and financial hardships of children.

CHAPTER 14

PREGNANCY

This is a section where you throw away all of the rules. Pregnancy is the state where the woman can suffer temporary insanity. Even she sometimes can't make sense out of her actions. She's having a cascade of emotions secondary to her ever-changing hormones. Because of all the influx of hormones her emotional "river", (see chapter 4 "The Digital-analog Male-female interface) is at flood stage, climbing out of the banks of normalcy. The hormone changes are normal and expected. That's why the typical alpha-dog rules and guidelines won't apply here. We've developed some "temporary" guidelines to help ease the pain of this process. This is definitely not an attempt at a cure but symptomatic relief at best. It's a time where the alpha-dog must be at his best to anticipate her needs and provide acceptable relief to her dilemma. This isn't a time to "kiss ass" and give up your hard found leadership. It is a time of accommodation, good planning and a prayer or two.

FETAL DEVELOPMENT, (thumbnail sketch)

It's best to have at least a working knowledge of the pregnancy process. If you know what's coming then you're not so freaked out. Pregnancy is divided into three trimesters, (1st, 2d and 3d).

THE FIRST TRIMESTER. The first trimester is the most important developmentally. All major organs and most importantly the brain and spinal cord are initially developed. Fucking up here can lead to anything from mild to major birth defects, (retardation, attention deficit disorder and autism are some of the few). They're volumes of research dedicated to pregnancy relating to food intake, drugs, smoking, alcohol and stress. Some research indicated that excessive stress during the pregnancy higher incidences of homosexuality then control groups. Apparently a study was done on women who were pregnant during the London bombings of WWII. This group had a significantly higher rate of homosexual babies than the un-bombed women. They concluded the rise in homosexuality was due to excessive stress. Why am I saying this? Well it's obvious that most fathers don't want their son to be a "rump ranger or a turd burgler" does he? Family reunions kind of sucks when he brings his "boyfriend". Is this research true? Who the fuck knows? But why take a chance? It's your job to try to keep the woman's environment as stress free and toxin free as humanly possible. The first trimester is so important. You must also abstain from alcohol, cigarettes and caffeine during the pregnancy,(they can cross the placenta and fuck up the kid). Even though you don't get her ability for multiple orgasms as she does you must feel the pain of giving up those things for the baby's health. The woman wants to feel like she isn't in this alone. We must do our part for the good of the baby. So drink Gin (it's hard to smell it on your breath), and drink your coffee at work. But cigarettes you do have to give up. A woman's sense of smell becomes significantly better during this time. Cigarettes will be picked up, if she doesn't smoke herself she very much could get sick form the smoke.

MORNING SICKNESS

During the first trimester one of the first and most frequent signs the woman might incur is the presence of "morning sickness". This doesn't necessarily have to be in the morning, but typically is. It's where the pregnant female has to "hurl" up whatever is left in her stomach from her meals. The process is simple, once pregnant the baby will cause, (through hormones) a slowing down of peristalsis, (the natural "squeezing" action of your intestines that moves food through your digestive tract. This slowing down is to allow for the absorption of more food and is considered normal so you shouldn't be too alarmed. This slowing down will cause the remaining food in the stomach to putrefy making her sick. If the hurling is excessive then tell the MD about it right away. Some remedies include eating more meals of smaller portions. But get a baby book for all the good tips.

Actions on the objective. The alpha leader should go into the bathroom with the female when she has to spew. You should do some sort of sympathetic action like hold her hair out of the hurl flow, help hold her stomach during the spewing process, give her a wash cloth when she's done or some other "I feel you pain" shit like that. But the key here is that YOU'RE THERE WITH HER! Remember postulate #1. SHE WILL FORGIVE BUT NEVER FORGET. Your act of kindness today may or may not be forgotten but your insensitiveness and "don't give a shit attitude" will definitely be remembered and cataloged for later if you don't._

Second trimester. The baby continues development and grows. Hormones continue to prepare the mother for the delivery.

Third trimester. The baby is pretty much developed and all it does is grow and mature. It's preparing for life on the outside. Typically your female's belly will grow more than any other time. She will also be dead dog tired all of the time. Her heart and organs are supporting two lives. Expect her to tire easily and help her at every opportunity.

STRETCH MARKS

As we said above the third trimester will allow the baby to get larger in preparation for life out side of the womb. The woman's body has to accommodate the growth. Some women's bodies do this well ... others don't. The rapid expansion of her belly can leave some women with the presence of stretch marks. This is a "body image" assault on her "chi" and the potential for her to freak out is high. Even though she knows that this can happen she hopes that she'll be one of the lucky ones.

Actions on the objective: Play down the stretch marks. Help her by getting some sort of stretch marks lotion to rub on her belly. NEVER, NEVER, NEVER point out her stretch marks to her. Don't stare at them, don't ridicule her about them and always lie that they don't turn you off.

ALPHA DOG LEADERSHIP

For our purposes the important thing is the mental/emotional changes that can take place during the pregnancy. The first change will be the hormone changes. These can cause wild mood changes in the woman. They can and will get very emotional. Don't take this as a mental condition that you didn't detect. This is a transitory condition and although not avoidable it can be dealt with. You don't look for a cure here. The cure lies in the delivery of a healthy baby. Pregnancy is like a cold, you treat it symptomatically. If she is suddenly sad you hug her and reassure her everything is going to be all right. If she's crying that she's fat or ugly you at this time reassure her she's at the most beautiful state she's ever been. Get her what she wants, give her lots and lots of Oprah type understanding and love. Expand the date nights to two a week, send more spontaneous flowers and make her feel as special as humanly possible. Remember our first postulate is especially important here, SHE WILL FORGIVE BUT NEVER FORGET. If you treat her extra right now the first postulate will work in your favor. If not it's almost like double jeopardy. The fuck you points are doubled.

Fat is a subject that we have vehemently strayed away from. Now you may comment on fat to your mate. You must lie tell her that she isn't fat that it's all the baby and you're confident that once she delivers she won't notice anything or words to that effect. Don't tell her you'll help her loose the weight, go on a diet with her or anything like that. Say nothing that will validate her fatted ness. General rules for this follows:

1) Be proactive. Tell her each day how beautiful she is. Twice or three times a day. Buy her flowers, get her treats that you'll know she wants. Anything but you do it first. Keep her busy with your attention so she won't have time to boo hoo to her self.
2) Take her on a walk each day for one hour. When you get home from work, walk her and talk to her. Remember no stress. It'll be time well spent and occupy her time in good pursuit. Remember you're the man the leader. Lead her to feel good by keeping her busy and exercise. When she exercises she will sleep better, sunshine will help promote good vitamin D production and help to keep some of the weight off.
3) Feeding. Keep the food healthy. If possible keep the food she eats healthy. She will undoubtedly want some shit food. Pregnant women have urges to eat the strangest stuff. Get it for her, and if she wants ice cream give it to her. She, for the time being, is the Princesses you're the supportive prince, (notice I didn't say servant).

Lamaze classes. This is very important to the woman. She is going through this and so will you. It's immensely informative about pregnancy and you will benefit from the closeness you two will share. It will also help you get closer to the whole baby thing. Men have traditionally been separated from this. Doing the coaching thing is kind of fun. Don't blow this off or make fun of it. Like the counseling, you take everything seriously. Don't hang out with the other expectant fathers who are cutting up or screwing around. Take your homework seriously do the breathing exercises with her on a regular basis. Remember postulate #1 SHE WILL

FORGIVE, BUT NEVER FORGET. The work you do here will have immense payback at a later date.

The delivery. If you have done your Lamaze classes well with her then she will feel more confident to deliver the bay without the use of too many drugs. Fewer drugs are better for the baby. She'll have pain but that's a small price for a healthy baby. I've been through three of these deliveries and the pain isn't that bad, (just joking ladies). Prepare yourself for what happens during the event so you don't get caught getting sick and or passing out. Remember you're the man, the leader you can do this. After the birth you will feel incredibly close to your mate. It will be a special moment for both of you. Enjoy this event there is nothing like it. Visit her regularly and of course bring her flowers.

Coming home. When you get home for the first few weeks you still have to baby her. She'll usually have been sliced from stem to stern from her episiotomy, (a cut they make so the baby doesn't tear the vaginal opening). Sex is out for at least a couple of weeks. She might want her mother to visit for a while. This is okay and you must not say anything. If she doesn't like what you do just smile. The bitch will leave eventually. Once her routine is established you can begin to return to your old routine, which you will now modify to include your child. Sex. You probably will have been with out sex for a good month now. Don't be impatient right now. She might be very scared for her it will be like the first time again. If the doc has done his job right they usually stitch up the pus a little tighter than previously. This is called a "love knot" and if done properly bring you back to at least your baseline opening. If not sex could be like throwing a broomstick into a gymnasium. Whatever happens you must not let her think anything has happened to her body except good stuff. Remember the connection between her self-esteem and her performance, especially in bed. She is particularly venerable now. Lies are very much accepted here. Some good actions are:

1) As with the pregnancy. After a small time period start to exercise. Initially disguise this as the walk. Gather up your child in the stroller and when you get home from work at night take her out for a walk. She will love you for it and you will reap the benefits from this. When people exercise they always feel better physically and mentally. Her weight will start to come off and she will have an increase in self-esteem. That's always is a good thing.
2) Continue the date night. You round up the baby sitter, get the reservations and take her out to dinner and a show. Show her that her life isn't over because we have children. Self-esteem, self-esteem and more self-esteem.

3) Buy her clothes. Take her shopping. Women with a new outfit will make her feel better. True it might cost some cash especially with a new child, but the benefits will outweigh the cost by far. You want to get her on the healthy thought process as soon as possible. Keep her away from what Zig Ziglar calls "Stinkin thinkin". Besides if you take her shopping it can save you a lot more money then if she went with her friends.
4) Go out with couples that have new children. There's always safety in numbers. Women (even though you do the good thing) will need the company of other women who have gone through the same thing recently. It's always best to associate with couples where the other woman is fat and their husbands are fuck sticks. This way she'll feel better about herself and appreciate you much more. Avoid the hot looking Momma. If your mate is battling with the fat thing then avoid women who have conquered fat after childbirth like the plague. If you have a mutual friend that is hot, then start a rumor to her that you heard she already had liposuction or something to that effect.
5) Avoid the eye candy. Either recently delivered or having trouble with the fat thing, when out avoid looking at the eye candy at whatever cost. You will pay dearly and the sex, if you get it, will be shitty. The shot to her self-esteem is immense and irreparable. If you get caught at this then we hope you enjoy tossing off.

POST PARTUM DEPRESSION

Some women, (not all) can suffer from the "baby blues". This is caused by the shift in hormones to the pre-pregnancy state. She'll be happy as hell one minute then crying out her eyes the next minute. All of her fears, concerns and the fact that she's now a real live MOM are facing her now. There's nothing you did to cause it. It just happens.

Actions on the objective: This is symptomatic relief only. Hold her, (if she wants to be held), talk to her and just be there. She may make some outbursts, scream at you, but being the cool calm alpha-dog you take it in stride. Talk to your OBGYN, (pregnancy Dr.) if the depression lasts too long

This is pregnancy in a nutshell. It's a time of miracles. It's also a time of trial and tribulation for both parties. This is where the alpha-dog is on high alert for her needs. Quick identification of her needs and wants will further increase her trust in your abilities and leadership.

CHAPTER 15

MARRIED LIFE A.C.

At this time you have made the ultimate sacrifice and not only did you purchase the cow you have given her copyright status and royalties for future endeavors. Since the birth of a child you have become permanently attached to the female financially, emotionally and spiritually forever. Regardless of a divorce you'll be bonded by children and/or the courts. The financial portion will eventually end but the other two will endure forever bonded by your children. The female you have now bonded with you own the good, the bad and unfortunately sometimes the ugly. Hopefully you have chosen well and you'll have an easy journey from this point. Don't have a false sense of security. The chores you have ahead of you are still arduous and many pitfalls could turn a good woman into a seething beast. This is not a chapter on the care of babies. It's a chapter on how to maintain good female management during this trying time. The baby tips presented are those that point out a potential pitfall for the man. It will detail your increased support to the female while, hopefully, not loosing the alpha leader status you have established. You will loosen the reins slightly but still maintain control throughout this operation.

AT HOME WITH BABY

By now you have gone through the birthing process and have just come home with the newest version of the union of you and your mate. This is your immortality, the little snip-it of your genetic material that will hopefully go forward into the future. Your attention to its health and mental stability will be judged by his contribution to the world. You'll either be a hero or a goat depending on your child's performance in life.

As with any good operations plan you have to assess the mission:

1) First time mother. The first one is always the most terrifying for both Mom and Dad. Unless she's been the oldest child and has had extensive experience in dealing with small children you have a female that is probably terrified at the aspect of caring for this new life. This means you as the male leader must have your Captain Kirk hat on ready to alieve her fears and give her the emotional sustenance she'll need to survive. The good news is that with each successive child the emotional trauma of the birth/home coming process lessens. Always bear in mind postulate #1 "SHE WILL FORGIVE BUT NEVER FORGET". This is especially true and acts of commission and omission in her great time of need carry double and triple word scores. So pay very close attention to her needs.
2) "Working mother" vs. "at home mother". Two concepts with two plans to be developed. Dependent on which one you have chosen. Aside from extraordinary circumstances, you should have planed for this contingency during your initial planning process. Either way is okay especially if you have planned for the non working mother. If not you as the leader must get out the plan and begin to re-work the essentials. THIS IS NOT THE TIME TO INCLUDE THE FEMALE IN THIS. She has enough to worry about. You can present it to her later.
3) Proximity to mothers. This is also an important consideration. Once the young mother is home she will quickly be inundated with the tasks of life with children. Having another set of hands to help, (especially a woman's) is a Godsend. It will ease in her transition and give her the necessary sleep that plagues all parents.

GENERAL CONSIDERSTIONS

Here are some generic/widely accepted considerations that the man must allow for:

1) She'll be dead tired. Actually both of you will. Babies sleep intermittently all the time. They eat, they shit and they eat and they shit. In between they like to be held. This doesn't correspond to the normal adult's concept of sleep/awake routine. So you must

accommodate and be supportive of the inevitable disruptions. Your support is needed if for nothing else symbolic gestures. Remember postulate #1 "SHE WILL FORGIVE, BUT NEVER FORGET". This is public relations at its best. You will need to "feel the pain" of her plight regardless of the loss of sleep you get. You are the man, you take the lead. Don't give her the reason to look at you with disdain and watch you sleep uninterrupted while she takes care of the baby you fuck stick. Even if she's breast feeding, you get up and get her a glass of water or some other stupid symbolic shit like that. You're the man be the man!

2) She is mentally, emotionally and physically exhausted. She has no reprieve from this either. Genetically and culturally she has the duty of the caretaker of the child. If she works she'll have to come home and take care of the child. If she doesn't work she has to take care of the child ALL DAY LONG. Extreme care must be given to the situation and anticipation of needs and wants must be met without demand.

3) Don't force sex. You should have had sex already but remembering the above you have to allow for her to signal when she has the energy and desire to dedicate to sex. She will be bearing the brunt of the child duties and she's probably not used to such physical and mental expenditure. You must allow her to have the necessary rest to function. Be kind, be gentle and offer touch as much as she wants. At this time never force the sex issue. Remember postulate #1 "SHE WILL FORGIVE, BUT NEVER FORGET". Today's poor pitiful fuck you bullied her into will be logged in that stamp book for future use.

4) She might be ashamed of her body. Once she gets done with the delivery and gets home she's probably going to be a little bit "saggy" and her tits are probably going to be tight if she nurses. She's going to feel all out of proportion. Expect this and don't bully or shame her into sex. Give her time and she'll come around. When you do have sex she might be possibly larger in a particular area. Don't be shit stupid and make any comment on it. Especially if you really like her big tits. When she stops breast feeding they're going to shrink and she'll fell inadequate. Enjoy the view and say nothing.

5) Have mother will travel. Don't bitch at the thought of "her mother" coming to visit. Pay for the travel and encourage her to stay as long as she can. You should be kissing her ass for taking the time to help. Having "her mother" to help, (depending on

their relationship) can garner you many points for future use. She will feel at ease having her mommy there and thank you for the thoughtfulness. Note: if her relationship to Mommy dearest sucks rethink the situation. Offer it up to her and let her choose you will get the points for consideration.

6) Consider maid service. If you have a working wife then you should consider obtaining the services of a maid/cleaning service for a couple of years. They don't live there they just come in and clean the house twice a week. This gives Momma chance to relax from work, play with the baby and give her energy to play with you in the sack later. If she's dead dog tired from work, housework baby, and cooking, sex is going to come in last on her "to do" list. Again she might do it, but she really won't want to. Do we want this kind of sex that deteriorates into rubber doll sex? This is your choice of course. If you don't have maid service suspend the first three months of household duties for the woman. Bring home carryout and drop off laundry for the female. You want to ease the burden as much as possible. NEVER DO HOUSEHOLD DUTIES YOURSELF. This is a classical error for many men. Contract out all household duties. If she sees you performing these duties it creates precedence for future negotiations that women are famous for. If forced to perform these duties you must do the guy thing… fuck it up. Don't worry; the majority of men don't have to work at this. Women will typically never be happy with the job men do on household duties. It's a wifely pride that they feel no one does it better than them.

    1) Date night. More important than ever. If you have the "Moms" helping out they will be familiar enough to provide a "night out for the "new Mom". This will be important in getting her out of the "Mom stage" and into the dual role of "Mom/wife". She will desperately need some time away from baby and the house to remind her that she has a life of her own. Establishing her as a creature that can have fun will pave the way for you and her to "have fun" in other ways like sex. The next logical step will be the "Saturday night getaway". About six months get her out for a night away. This will help both her and baby. The baby will get used to not having Mommy always near and train it to allow Mommy to leave for short periods of time. There's nothing worse than having your child demonstrating an encephalic scream worthy of

a Freddy Kruger film when you try and go out on a date. This WILL put a damper on the evening and is easer to start now while the child is young rather than later.

ALPHA DOG LEADERSHIP

As we said earlier don't wait for the woman to tell you what to do. That's why we're writing this book. So you'll KNOW what to do and do it before she "directs" you to do so. That's called leadership asshole. You do what has to be done with out anyone telling you. So what about all this "helping out". Does this damage the Alpha Dog leader? No if you are the one who decided it you're still in command of the situation. Now you are going to loosen the reins some but what you must understand is that the reins are still in your hands. You loosen them to allow her more latitude but your leadership won't allow her to run the show. She might feel "empowered" since it was her body that created life.... blah, blah, blah.... so don't give her any opportunities to give you "direction". Anticipate, anticipate and anticipate.

Example: Your wife is home with the baby and you have made the decision early on to help out. Like any operation you institute the five problem solving techniques:

1) Assess the problem. Take a moment and talk to the new Mother what are her needs. Adjust your plan to take into consideration her perceived needs. Anticipate what might be other needs she didn't mention. Close the loop on any ideas that are still open.
2) Make a plan. After establishing the needs devise a simple plan as to what you should do. This doesn't have to be fancy; a simple list of chores will suffice.
3) Implement the plan. The worlds best plan won't do shit if you don't put it into action. When doing this implementation makes sure she knows you're doing it. This helps later in the judge's arena.
4) Supervise the plan. As your implemented plan unfolds you will undoubtedly have to adjust fire for unexpected events. You have to remember your dealing with a woman and the propensity for unreasonable change is high secondary to hormones.
5) Evaluate the plan. After completion of the plan you need to evaluate it for the results. Did it relieve the mother's work load? What was its cost? Can it be repeated for future events or was it a "one time" plan.

Using these five steps you can retain the necessary leadership. Simply having a plan and a system for evaluation will place you leaps and bounds ahead of the typical man. The biggest threat to the man is unmet demand. Through your previous dealings with the female she has probably leaned to trust you and not challenge your authority. Remember to do a new "mental snapshot" after significant emotional events and reassess. Be sure to consider the speed of her "emotional river".

WEIGHT LOSS

As stated in earlier chapters weight is on the top of the list for women with respect to self esteem, self worth blah, blah, blah. THIS IS NOT THE TIME TO INSTITUTE WEIGHT CONTROL PROCEDURES. The woman is maxed out with the new mom thing, lack of sleep and returning to work looming on the horizon. You would be shit stupid to attempt to throw another rock in her back pack to carry at this time. Your goal is to lighten her load not pack her up. If you have chosen correctly, then she will be a self starter and generate her own weight loss program. Remember what we said about breast feeding earlier, it takes 1000 calories per day to generate breast milk. So suck away those calories junior. Refer to the weight loss section of the pregnancy chapter. Weight loss procedures may be started somewhere in the third to sixth month of home stay.

DATE NIGHT

It's important to reestablish date night as soon as possible. As we said earlier date night will give both of you the necessary reprieve from parenthood to endure. With out date night you'll quickly go into a rut and wake up a slave to the children. Dr. Shirley Glass, a Baltimore psychologist who specializes in Infidelity states that one of the greatest threats to marriage is the "child-centered marriage". Parents with dual careers often feel guilty about not being able to give time to them. In reality, one of the best gifts parents can give the children is to focus on the parental relationship; leave the kids with babysitters every once and a while. Have a life outside of the children.

If during the course of setting up date night the woman might not want to leave the children just yet. So a recommendation is to bring the date night to her. Set up the restaurant at home, get a babysitter and have the baby sitter watch the child at your house with you there. Then you serve a wonderful "take out" from one of her favorite restaurants. Get out the candles, the wine, (yes she should be able to have a glass at least when in doubt call your doc) and some soft music. BIG POINTS FOR YOU TODAY. You will be using postulate #1 to your advantage. And you should have some fun doing it. Note: Don't watch sports ass hole. It will devalue the entire operations. It's her night so become the supportive (not doting) husband.

RETURN TO WORK

Mom's first day back to work. If your plan calls for Mom to go to work somewhere between six and nine weeks she has to go back to work to work. This will really suck for Mom. Tremendous guilt, sadness and heartache can be felt by the female today. Review the females' ongoing conflict regarding career vs. motherhood. Remember postulate #1 SHE WILL FORGIVE, BUT NEVER FORGET. Plan ahead and schedule the day off of work, (wink, wink, nod, nod). Take her to work and allow enough time for her to cry and do all that sad shit that women have to do. You might want to take baby and her to lunch that day. This depends on how well she and baby did at the initial goodbye in the am.

Fuck It. Some mothers simply say "fuck it" and quit work. Now this is fine if you have won the lottery and are independently wealthy. But if you're like most couples you live at the maximum of what two paychecks buy and if she's heart broke you could be on your way to a severe financial fucking. If she's too distraught then back pedal in your plans and allow her the time to play Mommy dearest for awhile. Either way you're caught in a catch 22 situation. If you force her to stay at work you're a fuck stick and according to postulate #1 SHE WILL FORGIVE BUT NEVER FORGET, you're really most sincerely fucked because this is one of the super bowls of emotion for women. Anything bad that happens to this child will be your fault because you didn't allow her to stay at home and take care of the baby. If you have an emotional mate you should anticipate the potential for her not going back to work. Shit happens so don't box yourself in so tight financially that you couldn't do without her income. This is a good rule to live by anyway. Always make a woman's income supernumerary, (this means you really don't need her income to survive).

DAY CARE

This is a difficult subject for the baby books. Since we're not writing a baby book we're relieved. We do make the recommendation to research and study some child developmental books dealing with day care selection. Remember that your child is going to be principally cared for by someone who makes minimum wage (and probably can't get work elsewhere). Also as caring as this person could be, they still won't give the love that a natural parent would give. There are exceptions but you don't want to base your life on that fact. Your child will be exposed to all of the childhood diseases in your community since many parents can't afford to stay at home with their child when they're sick. So careful research and selection of a good daycare is mandatory. The key point is that the man should be intimately involved with the mother in the selection of the day care. He should also be there when the child is dropped off for the first few times. This is particularly hard on the woman and will appreciate your support. Actually this isn't a voluntary action. She won't tell you to be there but she'll want you to be there. You need to be there for her support and the "sharing of the pain" of her cleaving herself from her baby and abandoning her responsibilities of mother hood to a person who probably makes minimum wage. This is a little melodramatic but the chances are this is what she's feeling. You should act sad and forlorn because she is, if you don't you will be sad and forlorn later on when she's too upset to make love.

The man should also pick up the child from day care. This is another "sharing" method and will allow the woman to think she's not in it alone. It will also give the man some time alone with his child. For many men this is a foreign concept. Get to know the child's caretakers the program and progress the child is making. If you have made the decision to have a child then you need to help raise the child. The old saying I make the money around here doesn't work anymore. Children need your time and love. You can't package it or delegate it.

LIVE-INs

Some couples will have enough money to hire a "live-in" babysitter. The rich call them opairs, the middleclass call then "nannys" and the lower class call then nothing because they can't afford it, (I'm not trying to be a snob here just calling them like I see 'em). If you can afford it then this is the way to go. You have a permanent watch the kids anytime type of person. The downside is that you loose some privacy and healthcare for the nanny is a concern. Overall high marks for this because you have more control over the care of your child.

PICTURES

To Guys this seems like the most trivial bullshit ever created in the world. But to a woman it's manna from heaven. Guys just don't get it when it comes to pictures. Unless you're an amateur photographer or in the closet gay you can never appreciate a good quality photograph. They cost money and you have to make an appointment to do something that you could probably do just as well with your new digital camera. Give it up!!!! You have to get the picture. So to protect the alpha dog leadership principal when she suggests the photo op just say that's a great idea! And let it happen. You should be enthusiastic and supportive. This is non negotiable and in your best interest to do it.

1) The newborn picture. It's taken right after the birth in the hospital. This is usually expensive but if she even hints at wanting it you get it no questions asked. Never mind that you have just taken three roles of film of her shitting the kid out of the chute complete with after birth, cutting the cord and the special "bonding" moment of the mother and child. All captured so perfectly that you should get a fucking award. You have to get the hospital's cheap ass photo which would make a better mug shot than a portrait.
2) The "Family" Photo. Once home and the female gets settled in her environment you will be scheduled for the "Family Portrait". By this time you will have many many photographs of the three of you. It doesn't matter at all. She has to get a "professional photographer" to do the initial portrait. It will run about $100-150 for the pictures by the time you get all through. You have no choice in the matter you just have to do it. Get prepared to do one of these at least every other year if not every year. It's a girl thing so figure it into your annual budget. Note: Guys with other children should make every attempt to have the "whole family" together for the photo shoot. It helps with the family unity and eases the guilt you would have regarding your "other" children. Don't carry this into a major argument if your "other" children can't get to the photo shoot for an extended period of time, (greater than one month). She wants to document the production of your love together while the baby is small. Give into this and take another photo when your other children get there. By agreeing to this without an argument you save face and so does she. If the other children are there for the birth, get the family photo before she asks for it. Remember the five "Ps".

3) Holiday photos. Try and get the family photo during the Christmas holiday. It will avoid the extra holiday photo that some women like to get. If you have to put your foot down then this would be the one. You start this and their will be Easter, Thanksgiving, and Halloween. The way out of this is YOU suggest it, (and even schedule it). Then you're done for the year.

Note: Buy a good quality digital camera. The female with the first child will want to photograph everything the child will do, (1st crawl/walk/run etc). If you do conventional photography you will be very poor. Pay the initial cost up front and you'll save an enormous amount of money over five years.

HOLIDAYS

This is where it can get sticky, especially if you have parents that live far away or are divorced. You thought the demand of your holiday time was bad when you got married. Now that you have procreated you have no life at the holiday season. Its open season and the guilt arrows will be flying like the dogs of hell. If you're finally getting the hang of our book you will have already fleshed out a plan with the mate and your families. Although this doesn't get you out of the guilt zone, it will give you some protection and provide you with a framework for a fair distribution of the baby. Yes now that you have a sprout they don't give a shit about you. They want that baby! Some parents will stomp their feet or make a lot of noise and others will "suffer in silence" telling the female about their extreme pain and sorrow after the event securing a good reservation for the following year. Just remember that there is no 100% solution for this. Someone will be pissed and someone will be happy. Try for Covey's "win win" and hope that you can broker a deal that will suffice the majority of the grandparents needs. In town will be no big deal… Christmas at your house! Out of towners will have to be shipped in if possible.

SCHOOL

Parent – Teacher Conferences. It should be a given that you will take off, (if at all humanly possible) for the parent teacher conferences. You should be very interested in the educational and emotional developmental status of your child. Again if you took the time to have a child, then you must take part in all aspects of raising the child. Most employers with adequate notice will allow you to take off for an event. This will make your mate beam with pride because most fathers don't. They say they can't but when faced with the prospect of watching the Knicks play would gladly "arrange" the time off. So don't be a fuck stick, kids have parent teacher conferences at least twice a year. This isn't "rocket science" it's simply scheduling those events in advance.

Special Events. Every year a child's school or church has special events that center around the holidays. They have school plays, open house at the school and graduation ceremonies at the end of each academic year. Make your plans and schedule them into your yearly schedule. The look on your child's face will be worth it and the look on your face when you're having great fucking sex will be worth it. Remember when women feel supported, successful and complete they always will perform better. Leaving them to do it all by themselves only fills them with disdain and makes them a likely target for a hostile takeover.

SUMMER VACATION

Until the United States gets its head out of its collective ass you will be faced with the trauma of the "Summer Vacation". This is where the school opens its doors and the children are let out for the summer. We think this was started to allow the children to help out on the farm or some other shit like that. Regardless of the origin you have to have a plan in place to not only supervise them, but make a meaningful experience for them. Look into several camps for the children to attend throughout the summer. This is a much better prospect than having "Benny the pot dealer" give out free samples. It's much easier and cheaper to spend the money for a YMCA camp than to send your child to rehab. Stay involved and remember the five "Ps".

Family Vacation. This can "chew" up almost three weeks of their time. It can encompass a myriad of things. Disney World, National Parks and fishing are some easy ones. It is best to choose a mixture of vacation options for the children. A week at Disney, and two weeks touring some national park. A road trip is fun for the parks. It saves money for the air fair and gives you time with the children. We love road trips for this purpose. In order not to "overdose on the kids while in the car, we recommend you get a portable DVD player for the longer distances. This will give the children and you a break but still give you much more time with each other. Before you travel to a historic site, prepare a briefing for the children while at the home a couple of weeks before the trip. The briefing will enlighten the children to the significance of the journey and also heighten the trip by talking about it. Always try and do the educational portion of the trip before going to a "fun" thing like Disney. You can use Disney as a hostage for good behavior and compliance. Children like anybody else in the world need some motivation.

Parental Vacation. This is not normally done in the summer but we would like to talk about it here. Parents need to have a vacation for their own sanity. This will re-charge the mental batteries that have been long depleted during the work year. It serves as a reminder why we work so hard in our lives. Most importantly it reminds the parents that they, (as single entities) are a couple and why they got together in the first place. They need the time for rekindling of the childless years where they were experiencing the joy of love and limitless sex. As the man you need to include this in your annual schedule and financial planning. It doesn't have to be much, just a place to get away and relax. You might not get it the first year after children, but definitely in the second year. Adults need fun too. Hint: Cruises are fun, romantic, require very little planning and are relatively inexpensive.

THE COLLEGE FUND

If you are a believer of good financial management you should know that when you have a child you are morally and ethically responsible to get him/her as good as education as you can provide. College is to the today's 2020 child as was a high school diploma was to a 1960's graduate. So if you want your "Minnie Me" to dig ditches for the rest of his life rather than sit behind a desk and enjoy a better environment then do nothing. If you don't want that type of thing then you must start your savings plan now.

THE COUNSELOR

Weather you married or cohabitating a lot of couples will go into counseling for one problem or another. Even sucessful couples can have some un-resolvable issues. Going to a third party advisor isn't a "walk of shame". It all depends on how you view it. Having an idea of what to expect will help you endure the sessions. And at the same time get the most out of them. Hint: You might as well get the most out of them that you can since you're paying for them. Some basic rules are:

1) Take the counseling seriously. If she wants you to go to counseling then agree telling her that you think "we" should. Praise her on the idea but clearly let it be your decision. You are the man. When you meet the counselor be sincere, be participating and never, ever joke to her about the counseling. When you have to do things like

role-playing in front of her never be flip about it. We know it's so much shit. But it has to be done.

2) The counselor isn't "Judge Wappner". You don't go into the "People's Court" and state your case. It would be nice if that were the way but it isn't. The counselor isn't binding arbitration either. The counselor is a "communications specialist". The counselor is there to help you communicate your wants and desires to your mate in the hope of resolving your issues yourselves.
3) Always let the female pick the counselor. This is smart business because she will feel more comfortable. She will probably pick a female and you can rest easier. You don't think that you would have an easer time, but it's true. If you had a male counselor the male has a terribly hard time being unbiased with you. Remember: Postulate # 11 "WOMEN ARE THE VICTIMS OF ASSHOLE MEN AND OTHER MEN ARE THEIR RESCUERS". The woman counselor has an easer time with feminine tricks.
4) If you get a "homework assignment", just do it. Remember Postulate #1 : SHE WILL FORGIVE BUT NEVER FORGET. Besides if this works then you don't have to give the woman ½ of your world. Trust me this is by far easier to do this. Especially when the stakes are so large.
5) Never bitch about the money. If you bitch about the money it costs to go to counseling, then she'll only view you as a cheap son of a bitch who will say anything to end the high priced help. Look at the bill and swallow it whole.

For the woman to go to counseling is serious shit. Women typically don't like to air their dirty laundry, (especially in front of strangers). They have the tendency and would prefer to live in denial. But if their world is in such a shit they can't wicker the lie that it's all right anymore they go to get help. It doesn't matter who's at fault. Women get their "chi" all fucked up any place or by anyone. The issue is that you're the "bill payer". You're stuck trying to fix this shit. It may not be your fault, but **you** are responsible. This is your "wake-up call" Skippy. Fuck this up and you're in divorce court.

CHEATING

This section is most important overall in the married section. It will be likely that when married you and your wife will have the opportunity to cheat many times. It is the consensus of the writers that this is the most shit stupid thing that you could do in a marriage. Reasons are:

1) It ruins the sanctity of the marriage. Regardless of your religious preferences if you break your bond with your woman you'll never ever get back to the state you were once in. This is regardless if you're caught or not. Sometimes she'll "know". Women are very empathic. They can sense things like cheating or to a lesser extent a "disturbance in the force". The force being your attitude toward her and or life in general. They're typically not creatures of change but they can sense change in someone close to them.
2) You can get caught. Usually when women catch men "in the act" of cheating they haven't caught them with a wet dick. They've caught them on a date or situation that would indicate sex has happened, (wither or not it has in fact happened, to her it did). Once that happens you're so fucked. It'll also cause you to loose the moral high ground and the alpha leadership. Moral high ground is important when divorcing. You'll have mud slung all over the place and you don't need actual facts for the judge and more importantly the kids. Or she can forgive you. Remember POSTULATE # 1, "SHE WILL FORGIVE BUT NEVER FORGET". If she does forgive you your life will be a living hell from her mistrust. You'll have to account for all of your time from point to point. It will take years for her to get over it enough to give you trust and decent sex. Unless she does the "grudge fuck". See sex chapter.
3) The woman can turn you in. Take a look at the recent legal activity from a popular basketball star caught in the act by an accusing woman. He escaped jail time but now there's a civil suit, damages. Legal fees, lost advertising contracts etc. etc.
4) Women who would cheat with you will undoubtedly cheat on you. This is true to a very large extent. I suppose that there are exceptions but they're dumb asses and you don't want to be with them for long. Most women who are accomplices to a cheating man have many issues. You couldn't even begin to sift through them. Many times they paint themselves as a VICTIM of an unscrupulous fuck stick. Don't fall for the vortex of the victim in a cheating woman. If she doesn't give you pussy or just plays kissy face she just wants the added attention of you and it leaves you out in the cold possibly damaging your relationship further with your wife. We call this the "cheat tease" because the only wet dick you'll get is in the shower.
5) Women who are married and cheat on their husbands are especially dangerous. Run away quickly for your life. As above, but to a

greater extent. The woman who would break her bond with her husband and be an accomplice to you in breaking your bond to your wife has no moral value. She has extensive issues, is amoral, and should be avoided at all costs. What makes this even more dangerous is that most of these women are acquired in the work place. This is shit stupid and breaks so many rules and postulates you would be considered to have a death wish.

6) You could get the whore pregnant. There's a great avenue. Knock up a whore and pay twice the child support. This has happened to guys in the past. Please don't think that your dick is so great that you can find happiness with it.
7) Your whore could want, (or hate) you so much that she calls your wife up and confesses it all to her so you can be free or punished, (gulp).

Now having defined all the "downside" of cheating we feel compelled to give advice if you're hell bent on cheating or a low rent fuck with no self-control.

1) Get out of it. If at all possible extract yourself from the situation. If you haven't been discovered yet you will. Eventually most men who cheat and get away with it will grow tired of its allure. The problem is if the other person is happy you're okay. If not then she might want to keep you around. Or if she wants you fulltime she just might let it slip out that you have been screwing her to someone who will blab it all over your world. Then you're fucked.
2) Never get complacent with your security. Successful cheaters are Paranoid, type A personalities. You have to be anal with the cheating security. Women are very easily prone to relax. You have to be vigilant and definitely the leader here. Don't go to the same hotel more than twice. Don't eat out at a restaurant unless it can be clearly a "business" lunch. Never show public affection, and never call each other at the home are some of the easy ones to figure out.
3) Never fall in love with your whore. Many times the lust and excitement of a cheating engagement bleeds over into your life thinking you're in love. You might be if monkeys flew out your butt. But typically the two people get caught up in the moment and their life is so miserable at home they think they're in love. Well fucko that's not the way it works. 99.99% of the time it doesn't happen that way. You get divorced, she maybe gets divorced and you take up in a relationship. Eventually the lust wears off and

you're faced with the burning question "what did I see in this bitch anyway?" You also have to live with your personal shame for quite some time.

5) Never, never ever admit to the guilt of an affair. Even if you were caught with a wet dick on the front lawn of the white house, (Or in the Oval Office with a cigar) never admit guilt or confess. Confession is a selfish act done by one-way personalities who at the expense of others want to feel good about their particular sin. If you have to confess go to church and confess to a priest or a pastor, they're trained for this and won't be all fucked up when you tell them this.

That's that regarding cheating. If you didn't get the hint during this section then we will rephrase it one more time. If your marriage is shit then you must do the honorable thing... get out. You see when you cheat you mostly dishonor yourself. It will infect your self-esteem and affect you in all that you do. You will also be doing your mate a service by allowing her to get over her pain, find a new man and maybe find happiness, (with ½ of your world). The up side is that if you do divorce then you won't have to wake up each morning, look into the mirror and say "good morning Mr. Fuck Stick". If you think you're one of the smart ones and not get caught in a long-term cheat you might be. But the odds are against you on that one. This is the time and place where your only option is to do the right thing.

CHAPTER 16

DIVORCE

DEATH OF A COMMUNITY

Divorce in General

The decision to obtain a divorce is not easy. What you are about to embark upon is the most significant financial and emotional event you'll ever encounter in your life. When you go to court always remember that the judge will ask you one very important question. "Do you have a penis?" If you answer "yes" then everything will be your fault. Funny? Over reacting? 90/100 divorced men will probably tell you this is no joke. The more money you have the harder the divorce will be. Also remember this simple equation, "M=LI". Where M=money and LI=the opposing lawyers interest. As the money goes up so does the opposing lawyers interest.

Financially. As we said in chapter 1 divorce will leave you with one half of your joint marital assets. Joint marital assets are assets that are acquired during the marriage. This includes savings, pensions, property, (both investment and personal) and any other tangible item that can be sold or bartered. That's pretty much the norm for most of the states in the United States. If you have children then in most of the U.S. you can expect 20% of your net income for one child and 25% of you net for two and they usually have a schedule for each additional child. The cost goes up with each child and you're responsible for them until age 18. If they go to college you'll be responsible for ½ of the college expenses. Prior to starting, (or even mentioning to your spouse) the divorce, check out the upside and especially the downside with a qualified lawyer the local laws before making your decision.

Example: In Louisiana if your child is less than five years old you're responsible for 100% of his/her expenses until the child turns five, (that's typically the expenses your child has been used to living with). That means she can sit at your home raise your child and practice the perfect domino theory until your youngest child hits age five.

Emotional. When people divorce it ends a small "community", (especially when children are involved). Many experts say that divorce is equal or worse than death. Death has resolution your partner is gone, out of sight. You don't see your partner at the local watering hole drunk, hanging on, (probably going to fuck) on someone else. So the pain of loss is relived over and over and over. Eventually the scar heals but it's so tender it can be opened with a touch.

Children. With children divorce is even more traumatic. They say kids are resilient, they bounce right back. Well this is true on the surface. What happens to children they are forced to "CHOOSE" for the rest of their lives. Their love can't be a joint operation anymore. Mom and Dad was a unit, referred to in a collective sense. Now a lot of their emotions have to be divided. From this point on they will have to choose for all loyalties, emotions and love. If they love Dad too much it'll hurt Mom, if they love Mom too much it'll hurt Dad. Guilt will be always present on both sides of the equation. Remember they'll always have to live with this loss and you are a causative effect in their loss. One of the constituents of for children to develop into well balanced adults with good self esteem is stability. Having concrete values for them to build upon, (like Mom and Dad, home etc.). When you divorce a major concrete value, (home/ parents) are dissolved. It could tell them subconsciously that nothing is permanent; there is no safe haven in the world. You have been evicted from their world or something like that. We recommend that you should contact a child psychological counselor prior to initiating the divorce.

Since this is such a drastic step let's take a step back and look at your reasons for wanting the divorce. Some of those are:

1) I don't love my mate anymore. Well news flash stupid, if you have been married more than three years with anybody love is fleeting.... For everybody, (it's lust asshole). Real love takes longer to develop. You can have Cindy Crawford, Demi Moore or a host of other women and you'll find that love is still fleeting. A friend of mine had a saying regarding love "Think not that you

can control the destiny of love, for if it finds you worthy then it will surely control your destiny". Now that's pretty profound and sounds really really good in a bar to a girl you're trying to make her think you're a special sensitive guy. But once he got married himself he developed a new quote "Love is for two people who don't know each other yet". Much more profound, more workable and valid. Lust is what got you to the marriage point plus the first couple of years. Refer to "Love vs. Lust section. What keeps you together is commitment… nothing more. If you follow our rules and choose a woman who is more aligned to your life goals then keep her and learn to "re-love" her. It's a safe bet that you'll fall in love many times with your mate over the years. Seeking the "lust" of your ill-begotten youth again is a mistake and classified as "immediate gratification". Start down this path and you'll probably be miserable forever.

2) Your mate has changed significantly. When you choose a woman you have to accept the fact that through life changes and Significant Emotional Events she could "morph" on you. Again this reinforces our previous chapters on selection of a stable mate, but regardless if you followed our experiences/advice, you can still have a female that "morphs". If you have adhered to our book you'll have waited at least a minimum of three years prior to having children. Typically if a woman will "morph" she'll usually start the morphing in the first three years after marriage. You should have noticed something by now. Without children and an excessive buildup of assets you can unasss the marriage quickly without much residual financial and emotional damage. If you have NOT waited for the minimum time required and had children or she was a slow morpher, then you have to consider the change of your mate with much more discriminating factors.
3) Infidelity. Now we hope that you aren't so shit stupid that you are the adulterer. As we said before it would be the most stupid action of your life to do this. But I guess that's what separates the men from the boys right? If she is the adulterer then you have two things to consider.
    a. Can I forgive this woman? Yes we do believe in forgiveness. We encourage you to forgive her regardless of your feelings. Now why do we do this? For her? Not exactly. We do this for ourselves to gain closure. Why do we need closure? Because we recommend that you dump the bitch. We were tough on you if you cheated, so shall

we be on her. We feel that a cheating woman is even more significant than a cheating man. To a woman the concept of marriage and commitment is much more sacred that a cheating woman is doing a "double whammy". I hate to say this but when a man cheats typically he will cheat secondary to sex. Love can be there but it's the sex that drives him out. Women on the other hand cheat for deeper reasons. Reasons like love, self worth/self esteem, immediate gratification, lack of intimacy or a myriad of other things, sex is the last car on the train. So lets say the woman and man reconcile and try it again. The deeper reasons of the cheating are probably still there primarily because they're much harder to fix. If the underlying reasons aren't resolved quickly, the woman might be prone to cheat again or endure some emotional martyrdom for the sake of her family. If the cheating is secondary to a pathological origin then it would be hopeless to continue. Cut your losses and regroup for the next war.

   b. There is nothing else to consider. Sorry, if you're looking for a way to keep her and your dignity call "dial-a-prayer" and stop reading our book you pussy.

4. Significant Emotional Events. In the course of a relationship shit happens for real. The pain of the event has the ability to separate a couple and it's so strong it prevents the couple from returning to their baseline status. Some of these are:
   a. Death of a child. If it hits it can quickly bury a relationship along with the child. Get counseling immediately maybe or maybe not effective.
   b. Rape of the woman. When this happens it's disastrous and damages the relationship. Counseling is needed immediately and a long hard road is ahead for both of the couple.
   c. Rape of the man.... Yeah, nice try.

These aren't good reasons to divorce, they're just overwhelming reasons. Overwhelming reason and others like them overload the couple's compensatory mechanisms. Possibly they can't absorb the circumstances, pain or lack of control of their life and end up divorcing hoping that by changing something the pain will stop.

5. Poor reasons. Critical or disfiguring disease/accidents. It happens that when a spouse gets a terminal disease it separates the other spouse. The stress of an illness, disfigurement or other factors

lead to alienation of the affected spouse. In long term illnesses the unaffected spouse will have an affair secondary to stress, loneliness or sexual release. Anyone who would divorce their spouse in this instance is automatically placed in our "fuck stick hall of fame".

IMPLIMENTATION

You have weighed the facts and have made the conscious decision to pursue the divorce. Now is the time to PLAN for the divorce. Get a good book on divorce and do your research. As we said before, "proper planning eliminates piss poor performance", (the five "Ps"). So once decided start your problem solving formula and apply it to your current conundrum.

PROM AND THE DIVORCE

If Prom is pretty much about the dress, then divorce is pretty much about the lawyer. Your selection of a divorce lawyer is essential for your post divorce survival. The best bet is to contact several lawyers who SPECIALIZE in divorce. Specialists probably cost more, (especially if they're good), but when all you do is one particular function/aspect you tend to get better than the average guy.

A basic rule of thumb is the more net worth you have to loose, the more time and money you should spend on the lawyer. This is not a time to go cheap.

Now lawyers are creatures of consumption just like the rest of the world. They usually charge by the hour. So when you go in have at least a general idea of what you want out of the divorce. Bear in mind that you should have a "bottom line" for each area. Make sure your bottom line is reasonable. If the judge smells a fuck stick he can do almost anything. So areas of consideration are:

1) Cash. How much easily obtainable cash do you have on hand? You need some for the initial lawyers fees, (this is called a retainer and potentially you might be responsible for her retainer fees as well) and setting up your new domicile. Yes that's right asshole. You will probably have to move out at least temporary and probably permanently if you have children. Also you'll eventually have to share your liquid cash with your soon to be ex-. So remember the five "Ps".

2) Investments. What do you want, what do you want to give her? Anything you have invested in during the marriage is dividable. You have a lawyer to advise you but guess what? So does she!
3) Property. The house can go several ways. Usually if children are involved she'll get the house, (if she wants). Equity, (what you owe vs. what the house is worth) is to be divided. Sometimes the spouse buys out the other or they can wait until the house is sold and they split the equity. Sometimes the wife can have the house until the children are 18 and then be forced to sell to split the equity, (Your share could be a set amount determined at the time of the divorce). There are many ways to crack this nut. Just understand you can very easily end up with the shell. Investment property can be sold and split, (regardless if it isn't a good time to sell) or dolled out by negotiation or the judge.
4) Children. The rights for a man are pretty much set in the local laws. The national average is every other weekend, every Wednesday, alternating holidays, and so many weeks in the summer. Christmas is divided up in two and you switch every other year. If you live so many miles away you can get a longer summer vacation typically. If you're looking at getting custody the odds aren't in your favor generally speaking, (remember you have answered that you have a penis). You have to have a damn good case and then it's still iffy.
5) Retirement. Yes that's up for grabs as well. It get kind of tricky when both partners have retirement plans. But the judge will figure it out and is sure to make fair and equitable division, (like that's going to happen).

War Story. Bill was married to Jana and in the active military. They had decided to get a divorce. Their retirement plans were to be kept separate. That was until she got a lawyer who showed her a different spin. Since he was due to retire at 45 and collect 0-5 retirement pay, ($30-35,000) a year she no longer wanted their original agreement. She was willing to split both retirements. Since she was married to him for almost 20 years she got almost 50% of his retirement. He got half of her retirement, (not fucking much) payable at age 62. Do I need to continue? By the way he pays her this for the rest of his life, (unless she ups and dies).

SEPARATION ACTIONS

Telling the Wife. Once you have selected a lawyer, made your tentative wish list you are now ready for giving notice to your spouse.

This can be real hard if she doesn't see it coming. It's real easy if you're in an argument. "Fuck you bitch I want a divorce". You almost wish an argument to happen. But the best way is always the honorable way. Sit her down, be straight look her in the eye and tell her. One general rule: Don't tell her you've met someone else, (even if there is someone else). This is a "shit stupid" course of action. "It will awaken a giant beast and fill her with a terrible resolve" She'll have a cause and vengeance will be hers (and her lawyer's). In other words you'll really piss her off and she'll want to punish you. You'll have lost any moral high ground and she'll definitely tell your children what a philanderer, (fancy name for a fuck stick) you are. Your key theme throughout this entire operation is minimizing the shock to your children.

Telling the Children. The main concern is that you spare the children. If you can do it then you time the event when the children are away. Like summer camp. It'll give you time to get your shit out of the house and her to calm down. If at all possible it would be best to tell the children together and show then that you're both adults, (even though you don't act like right now). They'll cry and you both must be accommodating to that fact.

Keep the trouser trout in the weeds. If you left your wife for another woman you must have a clear understanding that while divorcing you are to have no contact with her. If you are discovered the damage to your divorce case can be irreparable. Opposing divorcing lawyers love to find the man whoring around. They can have a load of fun making you look like the "fuck stick" of the year in front of the judge. And they will if it will get them more stuff for their client.

Children. During your separation, it is imperative that you maintain a visiting schedule with your children. You're not divorcing them and they didn't do anything to cause the divorce. What do now will help minimize the emotional damage to them? It will also establish a pattern that you must maintain until they're grown. What you put into this could very possibly determine your long term relationship with your children. Even if you have to seek a temporary injunction for visitation, do it!

War Story. Another soldier had lived with a fat abusive wife for fourteen years. He was a good dad and had two daughters 16, 13 and a son 9. After many attempts of working out his marriage he eventually divorced. During the initial separation he didn't get to see his children for six months, (she kept them away). What happened during that time his two daughters were open to the mother's influence. What was once was a close relationship to them was replaced by hatred cultivated by the estranged wife. That was nine years ago. Despite numerous attempts his daughters have rarely talked to him, the oldest has gotten married, and (he wasn't invited). She had a child last year which he hasn't been able to see except from one picture given to him by a friend. The other daughter talked to him twice, (as a stranger), only his son accepts him. How could he have averted the hatred of his daughters? Who knows what six months of an angry wife's pain and influence could do to two teenage daughters? During that time no one defended him.

PRETRIAL NEGOTIATIONS

Many states have a "cooling off" period for couples filling. Texas is two months, Louisiana is six months. It varies state by state. We've discussed it earlier, but use this time to attempt a working settlement prior to your court date. Once in the pre-trial negotiation try to avoid entering into a argument that will give the lawyers a hard-on. Lawyers are people (barely), but they can get pissed off too, (generally at the other lawyer). Since they love to fight, and fighting makes them more money they can easy end up on auto-pilot and "duke it out". And why not? IT"S YOUR MONEY AND LIFE THEY'RE PLAYING WITH! Even if they lose the fucking farm and the kids they still get the same amount of money. Remember, the more you settle out of court the more you save in lawyer's fees. You also limit your exposure to the "whim" of the judge. He's the "wild card" of your immediate and permanent future. If you don't think that the judge's opinion of you doesn't count then let me sell you the Brooklyn bridge.

THE BIG DAY

THE LOVE/HATE Phenomena. When people get divorced we have noticed that they tend to hate those who was the initiator of the divorce action. We think that the love they gave in the relationship is closely to the level of hate developed in the divorce. So it would seem if your spouse gave you great love during your marriage she'll probably give you great hatred during and after your divorce. It is something you might want to be prepared for if you were thinking you guys could be "friends" after this was all over. Chances are she'll not want to be professional, congenial or anything like that. If you meet her out in public she might flip out if she sees you with another woman. This of course will be allowed and you will look like a fuck stick and of course she'll be a victim of your cruel emotional torments. Why is this....because you have a penis!

POST DIVORCE ACTIONS

There are some basic rules the newly divorced man should adhere to after the divorce. They are:

1) See the children… the sooner the better
2) See the children… Call them at least everyday. Everybody has 5 minutes for a quick call, (make this a habit).
3) See the children
4) Never have sex with the “ex-”.
5) Never communicate details though your children. This is an adult thing and children don’t need to be in this loop.

Initially she and possibly you will have tremendous anger after the divorce. Don’t let that get in the way of your relationship with your children. Give at the most one week without seeing the children. The sooner the better. Let them know that Dad didn’t divorce them.

WHEN THE GAVEL LANDS

Once the divorce is over you most likely will be pissed if you had to go to court. Most men feel like a financial rape victim. Don’t let your anger stop you from seeing your children. Never talk about the “ex-” in a unfavorable light. Wait at least six months before introducing your children to your new girlfriend.

Once again nobody wins in divorce except the lawyers. The biggest losers are the children. So focus on them. See them, do things with them. This should be your primary objective.

CHAPTER 17

END-EX, (END OF EXERCISE)

In retrospect women have been increasingly assuming control of their lives in some form or fashion for about thirty years, (1970-present). They have made leaps and bounds in social reform ostensibly to their benefit, (Equal pay/equal rights, single parenthood acceptance and "having it all" are well entrenched benefits for the women of the NWO). In doing an IPR, (in-process review) I still have some important questions regarding this major shift and its benefit to our society as a whole.

1. Has society benefited from the NWO?
    a. Divorce rate. Divorce is approximately 50%. This has markedly increased since 1960. No benefit here.
    b. Family unit disintegration. Back in the early 1900's when the Equal Rights Amendment, (ERA) was first introduced one of the main concerns was fear that the family unit would suffer from its enactment. We feel that the family unit has taken moderate to excessive critical "hits". Multiple extended family issues confuse and destroy traditional values, blended families, skewed loyalties between parent and child and spouse to spouse, resulting in a nation of children who hasn't the slightest idea of what a normal family was or is. Adding to the confusion these children are raised by minimum wage workers that staff the many day-care facilities. Children now take guns

to school and in conspiracy with others commit deadly acts of aggression, (remember Columbine High School?). This never happened in the 1960s when pistols and rifles could be easily purchased from a mail order catalog. No benefit here.

2. Are the women happier in the NWO than in 1960? Without directly polling the women in the US it's hard to determine. But looking indirectly we note the following:
   a. Walk through any self-help section of a book store and see the hundreds of titles of self-help books available to women. Why are their so many books? Why do they sell so well? Maybe because women aren't happy and they're still searching for some Betty Crocker "feel good" mental cook book that will be the panacea for their emotional conundrum, (problem). No benefit here.
   b. Depression. Approximately 1% of women born in the WWII era would experience severe depression in their lifetime. Between 12-15% of women born in the 1970's have already experienced at least one serious depressive episode. No benefit here.
   c. Anti-depressants. About 70% of antidepressant prescriptions today are given to women. In the 1960s you didn't see the large number of women taking "happy pills" that you see today. Why do we have so many depressed women out there? Why do they have to take these anti-depressants to "get through the day? What's changed between the woman of 1960 and the woman of today? No benefit here.
3. Women still get married. With all the un-happiness surrounding first, second and even third marriages women, (like men) still get married. They still have a dream that this is the way it's supposed to be to get true happiness. So like lemmings running into the sea they still walk down the aisle, make at least a temporary commitment in hope that this will complete them and end their unhappiness.

NO WAY BACK HOME

1960 was 1960. It's 2004 and we can't turn back time… we can only move forward and develop new strategies for survival. This is a book of trial and error, successes and failures. We hope that it gives you some new insight into developing your plan for a successful relationship. If this book helps one guy avoid a "never truly happy woman" then we would have considered ourselves and our efforts successful.

APPENDIX A

THE ROLE OF THE MALE IN THE NEW WORLD ORDER

With the rules changing in the New World Order, (NWO), the male must reinvent himself. Some old ideas combined with some new ideas to maximize his potential in the NWO. Since technology has "speeded up" the world the man doesn't get time to sit and "smell the roses". He's not allowed the "painful growth spurt" of fucking around for ten years. The old days a man could get himself a job at the "plant" work thirty years and retire to enjoy the "good life". In the NWO people change jobs much more frequently than ever before. Things have changed so much that the "vesting" statute for pensions have decreased from 10 years to 5 years. The NWO man must make his goals, decide his path and start to implement them on graduation if he is to enjoy a reasonable life with a reasonable retirement at a reasonable age.

When dealing with the female he must have "his plan" solidified and already set in motion. This will allow the man some benefits. One, he has a "map" of what needs to be done and how best to accomplish it. Two, women love men who have direction. It shows stability and purpose. Never mind the fact that she'll try and take you on a few scenic side trips from your plan. She is attracted to the fact that you have a plan and the dedication to that plan.

In order to help you with the establishment of a plan we have developed the following planning process. In the military we plan for everything. We plan for future operations, current operations, recovery operations, backward planning and a myriad of others. We have become very good at planning. We plan because we believe in the five "Ps". Proper Planning eliminates Piss Poor Performance. Like almost everything in this book it is not "cut in stone". You can use all or part of it for your endeavor. We only encourage you to HAVE A PLAN and implement it in your life. In-process Reviews, (IPR) are necessary to keep your plan adjusted to the outside events of the world. Your plan must be dynamic so you must ;

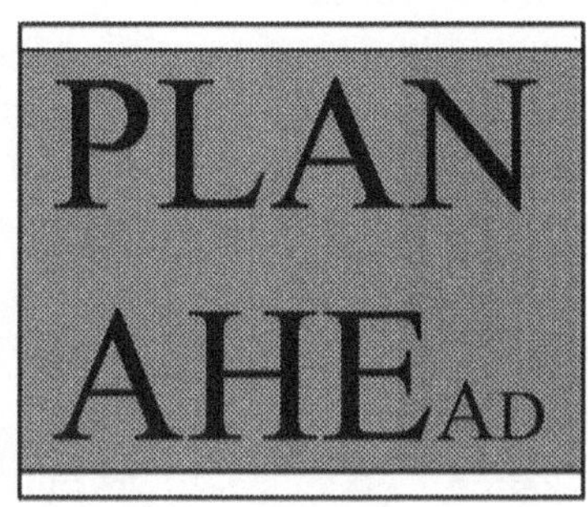

THE PLAN "A-WAY" FOR YOU TO PLAN YOUR LIFE:

Our intent here is to provide you with "a-way" or "a plan" to guide your life on. This is in no way the answer, in fact with life's strange turns, you could probably use your handy Captain Crunch Decoder Ring and get as close if not closer. Anyway, there are two inevitable events in life (outside of taxes), your birth and your death. Since these are predestined and there's nothing you can do about them, they will be preset and not part of the phases to your life. Initial State (birth) and End State (death) are managed by someone/thing higher than any of us. The "in-between time is in your control. Like the old saying goes, "If you don't know where you're going you'll probably end up somewhere else".

So your life, as we see it, will have 5 phases:

1) Phase I Education/Training
2) Phase II Initialization
3) Phase III Productive
4) Phase IV Zenith
5) Phase V Transition.

Each phase has a distinct function, the "long pole in the tent" and will (if managed properly) lay the foundation for the next phase. In the Initial State, you're a child so have fun! In the End State, your body is retiring so relax and look back on what will likely be a good life… if you have a plan. It is important to remember that a plan is only good at the time that you draft it. Forces and events shape your life and it will require to frequently revisit the plan to ensure you and your spouse are tracking with the "living document". The important thing is to have this starting point to adjust from because as you read this at 23 years of age, trust me tomorrow you will wake and be 40 years of age. It truly is amazing how time moves. Without any plan you will flounder and waste a great deal of time and money. We have more old friends that this last sentence applies to than all the other words above. It is important to establish a short list of key events in each phase that you would like to accomplish, together with a expected end state. Below is a brief outline of the time-line of your life:

INITIAL STATE

PHASE	BEGINS	AGE PERIOD
PH I Education & Training	18-20 yrs old	(18-27)
PH II Initialization	25-29 yrs old	(25-33)
PH III Productive	30-33 yrs old	(30-41)
PH IV Zenith	38-41 yrs old	(38-51)
PH V Transition	48-51 yrs old	(48-58)

END STATE

Each phase begins in a certain age window and has a time period, measured in years of age, for its length. Each phase overlaps at the front and back ends. This is not an exact science and is different for each person. Example, you may want to have children early and therefore have them grown and on their own earlier so as to allow you to retire earlier or to allow you more flexibility later in your career. You may not want to have children at all, therefore making the Initialization and Zenith periods shorter and the Productive period longer. You may want to surge your career efforts earlier in life and introduce a spouse later (35ish). This will give you a very brief Initialization period and a front loaded Productive period. This will also allow for a longer Zenith and possibly an earlier Transition (retirement).

1) PH I Education & Training: is the period when you obtain those skills that you desire or will need for your profession or career (productivity).
2) PH II Initialization: is the period when you launch your career or you begin In that area of the work force that you prepared for in

Phase I. Getting started in the productive (earning) phase of your life.

3) PH-III Productive: in this phase, you have established yourself in career or area of expertise and your ability to provide and earn is firmly established. It is the time you are climbing that ladder (whatever that ladder looks like).
4) PH-IV Zenith: in this phase all of your abilities have culminated; your earning potential, your knowledge of your chosen field, your physical health, your overall posture is likely to be at its prime. But, you are looking at twilight and must settle in making hard plans for it.
5) PH V Transition: in this phase you are scaling back your life and overhead. You are preparing for or entering retirement.

PHASE I (Education & Training Age 18-27)

At this point, you have graduated from high school and you will either join the work force, join the peace corps, join the armed forces, or go to some type of educational institute (college or trade school). We recommend college. You may not think college is for you, but give an honest try before tossing in the towel. We wish to make some points here regarding this phase.

General vs. Specialized. In your education (college), it is generally accepted that the more specialized you are, the more you can earn. However, the more general in nature your education is, it will allow you to apply for many different careers/jobs, but will reduce your earning potential. Why? Because "general" by definition does not set you apart from the rest of the applicants/peers. Specialized however, sets you apart and commands more compensation.

Choosing a career. In choosing your career, reflect back on your youth, and recall what your dreams were. This reflection can guide your decision making regarding career selection. You will need to prioritize your goals: money vs. geography (where you want to live) vs. mobility (willingness to continually relocate) vs. family (the desire for one). Perhaps the key in this phase is DON"T RUSH YOURSELF. You will make most of your key life long decisions in these 8 or so years. When selecting your major, plan for the long haul.

Research. You should be researching your career. Don't look at it what it's like now, but what it will likely be in high demand over the next 50 years, (with the peak occurring in 20 - 25 years). As always allow flexibility in your plan and application.

War Story. The current example is nursing. This is a specialized career, with a high demand, allowing for many different areas of focus, (ICU, Home Health, OR etc.). Employment can be found practically anywhere in the world and the pay is increasing because of a severe shortage. Nursing will likely be in demand for some time secondary to the aging of the "Baby Boomers", (a population segment roughly 3 times any other population segment in the U.S.). We're not suggesting that we all should run out and become nurses, but simply attempting to site an example of demand with a lot of versatility/flexibility.

Remember to play and travel as much as possible during this phase. This is YOUR time without family and job responsibilities. We don't recommend summer school, but rather take jobs in distant places where you can earn summer cash and experience some thing/people of different cultures (it helps trust me). If you think you will want to obtain a Masters Degree or PhD, then do it now! YOU WILL FIND IT VERY DIFFICULT TO DO IT LATER WITH RESPONSIBILITIES. Take jobs that work you at the bottom of your selected field. This experience in the trenches will pay big dividends in your career later. Remember: Any work experience, no matter how unrelated is seems and no matter how much you dislike it, the experience you gain will not be immediately evident, but all of it will serve some purpose in your future. For example, in the petroleum industry, if you choose to be a petroleum engineer, then work during the summers in the oil field as say a "roustabout" (the lowest worker bee on the food chain). The experience you gain will support your later decision making more than you can imagine as an engineer. You will understand what is happening where the "rubber meats the road" and will command respect of subordinates, which is a key to success. After all, the only real difference in careers is the technical focus. All other components are essentially the same no matter where you go: money management, people skills/interaction, illness, accidents, company policies, unions etc.

If you are attending a trade school, attempt to work in the field and travel as much as possible in the early years. Then settle into the school. You will need to go to work as soon as you finish your training and will likely not get a chance to travel.

Remember, DON'T RUSH yourself, obtain as much diversity as possible, don't ignore the dreams of your youth, and plan for the long haul. A list of your goals in this phase will likely look something like these:

1) Established your career preference
2) Established and attend the learning center/college of your choice (one that supports your chosen field best)
3) Completed all desired education

4) Accomplished a level of diversity in work and travel

End state: Selected and established career field, completed studies in preferred field, completed some travel and experiences in related field to ensure the chosen field is litegetemate. Reasonable idea of interest in life objectives and likely to be beginning or close to spouse selection.

PHASE II (Initialization Age 25-33)

OK, now you are a college or trade graduate and are ready to make your fortune. The early years of this phase will set the pace for your entire productive life so tread carefully at first. Here you are starting your career, you are more mature, and more stable. This phase is likely to be the phase where you get married (it should be). If you marry a women as old or older than you, it will likely work out very well. If however, you marry younger than you (younger than 23-25) then you are likely to be headed for trouble because she has not matured or has set about her career and become stabilized just yet. When this career settlement comes, you two are likely to see the future much differently. The closer to 30 you both are before marriage, the better off you will be and more likely to succeed as a couple. Don't forget the importance of insurance. This is an industry that is pretty much set so find the person or company you like and go with it. Some of the more affordable one is GIECO, and Farm Bureau to name a couple. Maintain this throughout your plan and remember to specify "replacement value" on contents and video your belongings

Children

Rule of thumb, don't have kids the first 3 years of marriage. In the first 3 years of marriage normally the "issues" surface, (see Married Life B.C.). If newborns are present you will not have the time and/or energy to address or fix these issues and the situation degenerates. If no issues develop in the first 3 years, then you (and her) have likely chosen wisely and your marriage will go well. At the end of the 3 years, is more than likely the best window for a child. Remember, you will measure your life by "before kids" and "after kids". You cannot begin to imagine how much your life changes when children enter into it. All that you took for granted: a quick change of Friday evening plans and you go to dinner, to a change in the weekend and you can sleep in late, to summer schedules (where the children are not in school). Everything changes. I'm a fan of children, but I know how important it is to at least attempt to prepare yourself for them and the subsequent changes.

Retirement

In this phase, it is time to begin your first retirement program. DO IT!!!!!!! A good rule of thumb is to place a minimum of 5% of your income in a program (up to the maximum allowable). A Roth IRA (or similar program) with a balanced portfolio is a good start. I realize that you will likely have some type of program with your job, but these jobs and companies come and go. Do not place all your eggs in your company basket. IF your confused, research the ENRON collapse during the George W. Bush's administration. The key to investing, that any book or firm representative will show you, is time. Money invested early in your life, even small amounts, has a much greater growth over the extended time allowed than larger sums "dumped" in during the productive & zenith phases (in your late 30's and 40's). Any reference worth its salt will explain this. By the way, your target for retirement is 55 years of age. A recent survey with Lockheed Martin, Boeing, and Ford concluded that for every year one works beyond the age of 55, two years of remaining life are traded. No matter how successful you are, PLAN TO PUNCH OUT AT 55.

House

Also in this phase you should buy your first house. The only acception to this would be the person that has prioritized mobility as one of the most important aspects of his life/career, in which case he should look at condominiums as transitional investments. The rule of thumb for high mobility persons is that you should be in one place at least 3 years to warrant a purchase of a condominium. Less than 3 years and you will not likely recoop your initial investment monies. If you project to be located in one place 5 to 7 years or more (which I don't consider that to be mobile), then buy a house! Rental expenditures is simply throwing good money after bad. There are many books and articles detailing the do's and don'ts of this, so buy the book regarding homes and re-estate. The other the reason that a book specializing on a particular subject, is that it is always important to get more than one point of view. In buying your first house, think small! Remember this is your starter house and will require room for you, the wife, and the new child. In most cases, these starter homes are best if they are "fixer uppers". In this case, you can rapidly develop equity with minimum effort and time. Money Magazine once published an article in which it stated that it appears that a persons 5th home is finally the one they want. Skill is required if you want to "up-scale" every time. I recommend up-scaling the first two houses following your starter home, then beginning to down-scale after that in order to set yourself on a comfortable footing for financial retirement. Don't get caught up in chasing the brass ring....IT IS OVER RATED!

A list of goals for this phase will likely look something like the following:

1) Purchase of starter home
2) Established in an initial investment program (outside of work)
3) Solidly established in the career field of your choice and producing
4) Married
5) One (at least the first) child
6) Evaluate your career path and make final determination it this is what you want (before you reach 40 and it is too late to change)

End state would look something like this: Living in starter home (location determined by either investment smarts, or education needs of young family), accepted in your field/office/job as grounded and a producer, paying particular attention to your spouse's needs and her "adjusted" PLAN, because it is in this phase that the two of you drift under the daily pressures.

Spouse

One critical point to make at this time in your life is that it has now become extremely important that you interact with your spouse closely and remain open to her needs/desires. It is difficult to explain this problem and impossible to explain why, but just as you have matured, so has your wife. Without realizing it, your goals and objectives have likely taken some subtle or maybe not so subtle turns in the last 8 or so years. Her goals will have likely taken some turns just as yours have. Throughout this phase keep an eye on her and remain a close part of her life (with date night etc, discussed in another chapter). At the end of this phase you will need to sit down with your spouse and re-look your (plural) plan. After this period of maturity/growth, either one or both of you will likely have changed to the point where you view your direction differently than you did fresh out of college/training. Revisit your PLAN together and adjust accordingly. The grind of toddlers and your efforts to advance in your career, not to mention her career, is likely to leave the both of you drained and at odds. Initiate a date night, at least once a month, and take a vacation without kids.

PHASE III (Productive or Main Effort)

In this phase, your setting the world on fire. You are moving forward on all fronts and your youth and education have manifested with a minimal level of experience, which has put you in the driver's seat of your career path. On average this period of 31-41 is when you have the energy to accomplish the most possible within any 10-year period of your life.

Spouse

At this point, if you have managed your relationship appropriately, your relationship should have transitioned from and earlier lust and later "fire fighting with toddlers", to a rich full love. Just as in the previous phase, it is critical to remain aware of your spouse and what she desires and fears. If your lives are taking a direction that she is not comfortable with, pay attention! Her career may have developed or is developing in a direction that will require the two of you to re-look your (the husband) career designs. It's a team effort, don't loose site of that fact. Guard against abandoning your goals in an effort to placate her desires. It is a two way street for her too! Also, in this phase, date night and dual vacations are critical. Schedule a date night with her at least once a month, and take one vacation with the kids, and one without the kids.

House

In the early years of this phase you should have sold your starter home and bought your second home. This home is likely to be the most important property purchase you make until you transition into retirement. If you are ever going to build a home, this is the time. If you build, do it in phases. This will allow you to maximize your money and build early equity because some of the finishing touches you can complete as you go and pay out of pocket. With this activity not under your mortgage, you can build quick equity. This option is not without its pain. If you do not want to bother with it, then a "turn key" plan is the one for you. In this plan, the General contractor and plans are selected and when it house is completely finished, all you are required to do is turn the key to the entrance door. If you go with this option, on piece of advise, is tear pictures out of magazines that accurately represent how you want the finished product to look. On anything from windows, to doors, to shutters, wall paper and shades of colors, a picture is worth a thousand words and cannot be explained clearly enough in plans. At the end of this phase, it is likely that you could be looking at the third home. The necessity for location for children and their education will likely dictate this buy (as it probably should). Resist the urge to up-scale. You will need the equity in 10 more short years. So go for similar size and cost but located and configured more to your taste and needs.

Children

I recommend that you complete your addition of children by age 37. At this point (if you had all of your children prior to 32), your early children are approaching their teenage years and (from their prospective) have forgotten more than you (the parents) know. They will likely be busier than ever before in sports, scouts, clubs, school etc. They do not yet possess the ability to drive them selves, and will require massive amounts of you and your spouse's time to meet all of the obligations just in transportation alone. Prior to this phase, the children were relatively easy to manage. Now begins their most critical window of development. As with the other sections of this chapter, I recommend a book on child rearing. However, I can tell you from experience that if you have provided a loving supportive environment for them in their younger years, then you've done your best. But, now is the test. In this phase of their lives it will be more important than ever for you to be involved in every facet of their lives. The types of friends and the interest that they develop, will profoundly shape their teenage years. STAY IN THERE…make the time. If you need it done around the house, either involve them and do it together (get them off of the couch or out from in front of the computer), or hire it out…but stay focused on them. It is also now that you and your spouse must maintain absolute open communications. The children will begin to attempt to "play both ends against the middle". It is critical that you and your spouse are seamless in your position regarding any decision. This will also unknowingly provide more evidence of a substantial family foundation and add to their security, even though they "hate" you at the moment. Its almost as if it's a big game and all are role playing to what is expected of them at that point in time. Stand your ground. Realizing that it is demanding for you and your wife, keep the kids involved in as much as possible. This will engage/challenge/develop them physically and mentally as well as reduce the idol time that tends to get them into trouble. The big events are easy to plan for, but it's the daily battles where the war is won.

Retirement

At the end of this phase, ages of 38-41, it is time to seriously look at your retirement program. By now you should have continued to add to the initial plan during the Initialization phase. You should also be moving forward in your company plan. In either or both cases, MAXIMIZE these each year. You will have good years and bad years but in the long haul, you will grow 7-10% and be where you need to be for retirement. It is also at this phase that you should consider additional investment opportunities, due to the fact that you have learned a lot more about the subject, and you have networked with people that can likely provide some conduit to opportunities. Also at this point take your first close look at retirement. Answer questions like: where do I want to retire, how much money will I really need to live on, what will be expected of me by family members (if anything) at that time, and what type of business or activity can I invest or engage in that will help reduce my taxable income at that time. This last question is particularly important because you will continue to be taxed as a retired person (with a few rare exceptions such as ROTH IRA's) but your income will be fixed with little opportunity to generate more income. This will likely be your last opportunity to launch any new initiative for retirement. Remember, the buying power of money is directly tied to time. The more time available, the more money can grow. So, after this point (early 40's) it is not likely that you will be able to generate any significant funds with the time remaining unless of course you purchase an existing business or win the lottery (or some similar windfall) and invest it all. Even then, their annual limits to what you can normally invest.

The following is a short list of goals for this phase:

1) Establish a solid retirement program
2) Settle the family (children) in a third house that is ideal for their needs
3) Integrate the children into enough activity for their well-being
4) Have re-looked your and your spouse's career posture
5) Form an initial plan for your retirement posture
6) Established schedule that maximizes time with kids

End State: Living in third house (not up-scaled) located for children and their education/social needs, having established a solid retirement program, having initiated the last of any major investments, having established the final phase of your and your spouse's career path, and set a schedule that maximizes your time with the kids.

PHASE IV (Zenith)

In this phase you are 38-51 and are beginning the steps of "down-sizing" to prepare for the Transition phase and retirement. It is in this phase that you purchase your last home (prior to your retirement environment). Children will either be teenagers in high school, or leaving home for their

PLAN. In any event your time with them is as critical or more critical as earlier with one subtle change. They are driving and don't need you for mobility. It is here that your career will be maturing and you will likely begin to consider how and when you will be throttling back there as well.

Spouse

Until now, you and your spouse have been moving at the speed of sound between careers, developing retirement programs, raising/ developing children, and attempting to stay in contact with each other. With all of the teenagers having mobility, you now suddenly have some of your life back (not too much due to the ever present need to keep tabs on the teens). Increase your date nights, but keep both vacations. The family corner stone is still crucial to the kids even though they seem oblivious to it. This is what is referred to as CULMINATION in military circles. The peek of your impact both in the family and in the work place is likely to be realized at this point/phase. Sit with your spouse and finalize her wishes/ aspirations for retirement so that the two of you are working in the same direction both fiscally and emotionally.

Children

At this point the kids are moving at the speed of sound but you are beginning to fall behind. They wouldn't have it any other way. They have their mobility and can completely fill everyday without you. Don't be fooled, they need your presence and the foundation of the family even though they appear to have no concept of it. It is also important to understand their interest and desires as they have developed over the past few years. You are now entering the window of college preparation. It is time to figure out what they "think" they want to study or do with their lives, and then help them (in some cases push them) in determining the best school for their interests.

Retirement

In this phase, you will likely not change too much on the retirement front. It is too late to dump large amounts of money and expect it to mature into large returns in time for retirement. Remember your target is 55. It is at this phase however, that you can and will likely identify any retirement "tax friendly" business that you will purchase or invest in (on this one, consult the specialist). Identify the location that you want to live while in retirement. It is likely that you will need to identify 3 or 4 locations. This is in no small part due to the kids and their locations. It is likely that you will want to be reasonable close to them. If not then it's a free fire zone and take your best shot. Price these locations and determine what cash flow will be required for this area and your desired standard of living. Earlier in this chapter, the term "retirement environment" was used. This simply means the location, type of home (structure-condo without maintenance requirements vs house with yard etc.), level of available disposable cash, types of services and activities that you prefer to have at your disposal etc that most closely matches your expectations. Now is the time that you nail down as close to possible this "retirement environment" for your planning purposes. As always, this is a joint decision and one of the last big ones you will likely make as a couple.

House

In this phase you may sell and buy one more house before your retirement environment. If this happens, DOWN-SIZE. The equity will be needed for any number of things such as: your daughters wedding (SORRY), your deposit on some desired retirement environment housing/ structure, or the last chance retirement business investment (not market type investment IRA etc.). In any event it may be more to your benefit to take out a second mortgage on your existing home and improve it in a way that will net more on the final act of sale (guest house etc.). With this option, be careful not to invest more money into the existing house, than the "comps" in the area will allow you to recovery at act of sale. We recommend that you stay put, and take a second mortgage for expenses or investments, as long as your surrounding area is improving and not degrading. The following is a list of possible goals at the end of this phase:

1) Steady state for all high school teenagers
2) Established final career plans for you and your spouse
3) Final determination for your retirement environment
4) Final decisions and actions taken and in place for Transition (retirement)

End State: Having set the final retirement plan into place. This plan includes the details of your retirement environment. Set in place the continuing/professional education institutions for the children, set environment supporting the children for completion of high school. Have set in place the final career plans for you and your spouse.

PHASE V (Transition)

It is in this phase that you leave the work force and move into your (plural) retirement environment. The children are out of the house, and you sell your current home for the move to the location and structure of retirement that you designated in the previous phase. The proceeds from the sell of the house will be available for this transition and or for the other daughters wedding (SORRY). Incidentally, don't forget that your life insurance policies accrue cash value that can be borrowed upon for such events as weddings etc., you won't need the money once it is collected! At this point you have a lot of time on your hands and no more significant investments are necessary.

Spouse

If she hasn't killed you or left you for a chip-n-dales dancer, your probably in pretty good shape as a couple. You will have enormous amounts of time on your hands and hopefully some cash flow from all the retirement planning to go places and experience things, where you didn't have the time or money before. Again, get her shopping list and go at it!

Retirement

In this phase, the only thing to discuss is the moving parts involved in the transition from the work force to retirement. You sell your house and all other holdings not key to your developed retirement environment and mass the cash to purchase those aspects of your retirement environment that you have identified. This act of sale and subsequent purchase is executed on or about the 55 year so as to minimize upheaval. If a "too good to be true" deal comes along earlier, then a couple years of renting will not be the end of the world, but remember that 1 or 2 year tax hit you will take. However, chances are that your interest on the existing house is so low that you probably are not going to get much of a tax break anyway so it may be a wash (either options outcome is the same).

Children

What children?

Goals and end state at this point is somewhat obvious. The years beyond 55 are considered end state in and of themselves and are available for what ever you want them to be. Good luck!

THOUGHTS FOR RECAP

-Don't rush your early education
-Have a plan
-When you meet misses right, brief the plan in nauseating detail

-Invest in retirement the moment you leave the learning environment and enter the work force

-Re-look this plan frequently, at least in the middle and at the end of each phase. This re-look must include the both of you

-Don't chase the brass ring, rather work towards your plan

-Ask around and get the best available references for: Managing a marriage, investments, insurance, child rearing, and retirement planning.

-This PLAN was intended as a "blue print" or "framework" for your planning. Read the books for the detail and then "plug" the detail into the framework or blueprint provided.

SET A LIST OF YOUR GOALS FOR EACH PHASE WITH AN END STATE CLEARLY DEFINED

APPENDIX B

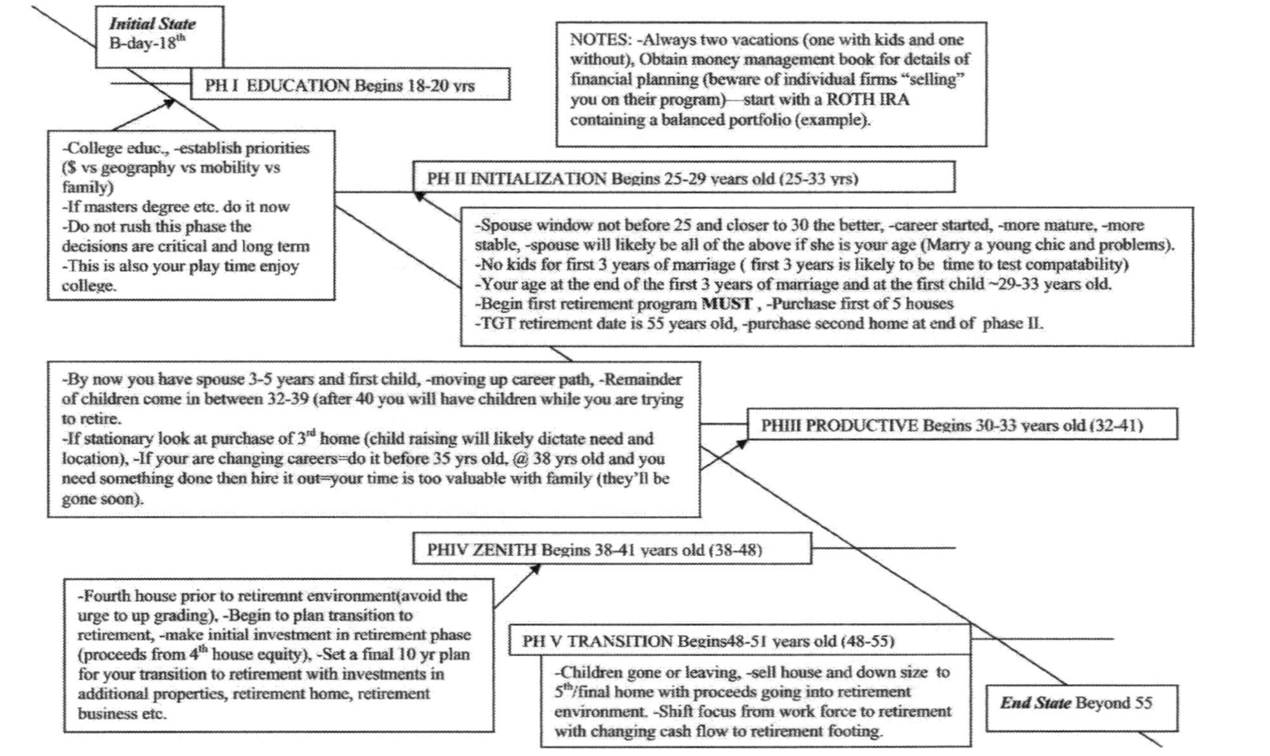

Initial State
B-day-18th
PH I EDUCATION Begins 18-20 yrs
-College educ., -establish priorities ($ vs geography vs mobility vs family)
-If masters degree etc. do it now
-Do not rush this phase the decisions are critical and long term
-This is also your play time enjoy college.
NOTES: -Always two vacations (one with kids and one without), Obtain money management book for details of financial planning (beware of individual firms "selling" you on their program)—start with a ROTH IRA containing a balanced portfolio (example).
PH II INITIALIZATION Begins 25-29 years old (25-33 yrs)
-Spouse window not before 25 and closer to 30 the better, -career started, -more mature, -more stable, -spouse will likely be all of the above if she is your age (Marry a young chic and problems).
-No kids for first 3 years of marriage (first 3 years is likely to be time to test compatability)
-Your age at the end of the first 3 years of marriage and at the first child ~29-33 years old.
-Begin first retirement program MUST , -Purchase first of 5 houses
-TGT retirement date is 55 years old, -purchase second home at end of phase II.
-By now you have spouse 3-5 years and first child, -moving up career path, -Remainder of children come in between 32-39 (after 40 you will have children while you are trying to retire.
-If stationary look at purchase of 3rd home (child raising will likely dictate need and location), -If your are changing careers=do it before 35 yrs old. @ 38 yrs old and you need something done then hire it out=your time is too valuable with family (they'll be gone soon).
PHIII PRODUCTIVE Begins 30-33 years old (32-41)
PHIV ZENITH Begins 38-41 years old (38-48)
-Fourth house prior to retiremnt environment(avoid the urge to up grading), -Begin to plan transition to retirement, -make initial investment in retirement phase (proceeds from 4th house equity), -Set a final 10 yr plan for your transition to retirement with investments in additional properties, retirement home, retirement business etc.
PH V TRANSITION Begins48-51 years old (48-55)
-Children gone or leaving, -sell house and down size to 5th/final home with proceeds going into retirement environment. -Shift focus from work force to retirement with changing cash flow to retirement footing.
End State Beyond 55

APPENDIX C

THE POSTULATES AT A GLANCE

POSTULATE #1 "SHE WILL FORGIVE, BUT NEVER FORGET

POSTULATE #2 WHAT YOU SAY AND DO CAN BE USED AGAINST YOU IN A COURT OF FEMININE FEELINGS

POSTULATE #3 "WHEN A WOMAN IS UNHAPPY SHE WILL TEND TO SHARE HER UNHAPPINESS"

POSTULATE #4 "WOMEN TEND TO LET SITUATIONS EVOLVE RATHER THAN MAKE A SOLID DECISION"

POSTULATE #5 "TWO PLUS TWO DOESN'T ALWAYS EQUAL FOUR"

POSTULATE #6 "FEMALES WILL ALWAYS TALK"

POSTULATE #7 "FEMALE FLAWS WILL TYPICALLY GET WORSE WITH TIME"

POSTULATE #8 "ONCE COMMITTED YOU ARE A WE OR US ENTITY"

POSTULATE #9 "WHEN WOMEN FEEL SPECIAL THEY PERFORM SPECIAL"

POSTULATE #10 "FACTS AREN'T IMPORTANT SO LONG AS THEY SUPPORT THE TRUTH"

POSTUALTE #11 "WOMEN ARE VICTIMS OF MEN AND OTHER MEN ARE THEIR RESCUERS"

APPENDIX D

THE NATURE OF MAN

Before we can attempt to develop successful survival strategies for female management, we must first understand ourselves. If we keep acting the same old way then we'll keep making the same old mistakes.

HERE I COME TO SAVE THE DAY!

This was the phrase that Mighty Mouse would sing while he was on his way to save his girlfriend. This episode she had once gain gotten her ass in a crack and needed Mighty Mouse to extract it. So of course he did and she nuzzles up to him in the end and everything is okay, (until next week).

As women are nurtures, men are rescuers. We can't help it. It's probably ingrained on our genetics somewhere to always protect the female of the species. This is typical since there are times when the female is very vulnerable, (pregnancy, raising the children.... shopping). There's a biological need to protect the female. It's like Geese flying south for the winter. Men can't resist a good "fixer upper". We have been taught this since our childhood. Why is this?

1. Boys don't hit girls. Remember that? It was ingrained in us since pre-K. We supposed to be stronger, faster, etc. so we shouldn't whoop their ass, (even if they whoop ours).

2. Good manners. Hold the door for the girls, ladies first, scoot the chair in for the lady…etc. This further reinforced men in establishing caretaker roles.
3. The media. The above items are important, but the real initiator of our rescue mentality is the media. Men have been selectively pre-programmed like Pavlov's dogs for this conditioned response. Some examples are:
    a. The animated damsel in distress. Here's the reoccurring theme that's just about everywhere in our world.
        i. Dudley Do Right. He had to save the fair Nell.
        ii. Underdog. He had to save Pure Polly Purebred from Overcat.
        iii. Popeye had to save Olive Oyl from Bluto.
    b. In movies the damsel in distress still played well continuing to indoctrinate us.
        i.. Luke Skywalker and Hans Solo had to save Princess Lea from Darth Vader.
        ii. George of the Jungle had to save Ursula from her ex-fiancée.
        ii. Tarzan had to save Jane.

This list can go on and on. We watched it from a toddler and even though we're grown up we're still watching it. What's more we like this shit. It fits in nicely with our testosterone. However while we were getting indoctrinated to be rescuers the girls were getting equal instruction on how to be damsels in distress, (read victims).

Actions on the objective: It's okay to be a "man" and save the damsel in distress. But you want to make sure that she's really in distress from an outside situation and not from something of her own design. Also make sure that she isn't always in "distress". Some women seem to always be in distress or conflict. Look for patterns of distress. Are you willing to put up with saving her all of the time for the rest of your life?

STRAIGHT OFF THE CUFF

Men have a tendency to talk "from the cuff". To say what they mean and mean what they say. We're blunt, to the point, decisive and we typically we don't change course without direct notice. I'm going to do this now. And then we… do it! This is sometimes in direct conflict with women and how they do things.

Actions on the objective: Learn to "keep your cards close to your chest". Be aloof and develop the concept of inaccessibility. Look for the trend in your female regarding her decisions. If she's a straight talker, (there are a few out there) then great. But if she's the typical female always step back and see the larger picture.

WERE STUCK

Lets face it were stuck in a particular mold and there's not much that can be done about. We just have to compensate and not let a female take advantage of the situation. We do this by recognizing the pathological and running like hell!

About the Author

Charles A. Becker has worked in all aspects of healthcare for over 15 years. He has done work in such areas such as crisis stablization, substance abuse/detoxification and emergency care. He is a career Army Reserve officer for over 23 years. He has recently returned from serving in Operation Iraqi Freedom.

William S. Brannigan Jr. is a career Army officer for over 18 years. His expertise is in operational doctrine and planning. He has also just returned from serving in Operation Iraqi Freedom and is preparing for a possible reactivation to Iraq.

www.ingramcontent.com/pod-product-compliance
Lightning Source LLC
Chambersburg PA
CBHW030259290526
45785CB00001B/143